PRIVATE PARTS

PRIVATE PARTS

A DOCTOR'S GUIDE
TO THE MALE ANATOMY

YOSH TAGUCHI, M.D.
Edited by Merrily Weisbord

DOUBLEDAY

NEW YORK LONDON TORONTO

SYDNEY AUCKLAND

PUBLISHED BY DOUBLEDAY
a division of Bantam Doubleday Dell Publishing Group, Inc.
666 Fifth Avenue, New York, New York 10103

DOUBLEDAY and the portrayal of an anchor with a dolphin
are trademarks of Doubleday, a division of Bantam Doubleday
Dell Publishing Group, Inc.

Library of Congress Cataloging-in-Publication Data
Taguchi, Yosh, 1933–
  Private parts.
  Includes index.
  1. Andrology—Popular works. 2. Generative organs,
Male. I. Weisbord, Merrily. II. Title.
RC881.T22   1989   616.6   88-30941

ISBN 0-385-26200-0

For my mother
and in memory of
my father

CONTENTS

CONTENTS

viii

10
WOMEN

11
HOW TO TAKE CARE OF YOUR PRIVATE PARTS

ACKNOWLEDGMENTS

I wish to thank my editor and friend, Merrily Weisbord, without whom my effort would likely have remained what Michael Crichton has called "medical obfuscation."

My thanks, also, to Patrick Crean, who did the final sprucing up of the manuscript; Dr. Hélène Rousseau, who contributed to the section on chlamydia; and Drs. Linda Kabbash and Norbert Gilmore of the Royal Victoria Hospital, Montreal, and Drs. Mary Henderson and Alexandra Beckett of Massachusetts General Hospital, who were of great help in the AIDS section.

In the early writing stages, authors J. J. Brown and Jack Kelley helped with constructive criticism. At this same time, Mike Rosenbloom's moral and practical encouragement were vital.

Over the years my professors and patients have broadened my outlook and understanding, and for this I am appreciative.

Finally, I wish to thank my family—Joan, Kathleen, Edwin, Jocelyn, and Carolin—for their patience and support.

INTRODUCTION

A generation ago, medical information was secret information privy only to members of the medical profession. And the members of the guild guarded their precious secrets with a proprietary interest. The secret they didn't want out was how little they knew.

The subterfuges employed were ingenious.

"There's no point trying to explain it, you wouldn't understand. You just concentrate on getting well and leave the worrying to me."

Or:

"It's a thingamajig."

"What?"

"What you have is a thingamajig."

"I don't understand."

(You're not supposed to.)

The keep-em-guessing principle was applied even to neophytes in the profession. When I was a junior intern in the orthopedic service, I wondered why we were bandaging a wound that had already healed. I asked the chief:

"Why are we applying wet sulfa dressings to a clean skin wound?"

His answer: "How often are you doing it, son?"

"Once a day, sir."

"Well, from this day forward, you will do it twice a day."

(End of conversation.)

Today, there are a plethora of "How to . . . ," "Why . . . ," and "Confessions of a . . ." type books on most medical subjects, but a popular book on the health problems of men's private parts does not exist.

The groin area has, for years, been taboo. This was brought home to me a few years ago when I instructed young medical students to pull the sheet down to the patient's mid-thigh level before they began the physical examination of the abdomen. By so doing, I suggested, the doctor shows the patient that he does not consider any part of the body embarrassing or sacrosanct. Furthermore, there are more health problems in the groin and genital area than there are a foot above or a foot below. And finally, pulling down the sheet ensures that this area will be examined and not passed over. Prescient advice, I thought. But I heard through the grapevine that I was out of line, that I was not respecting the privacy of citizens. Citizens yes, patients no, is my reply.

I see problems of the private parts every day, as I have for the past twenty-five years. As a young man, when I qualified as a surgical specialist in urology, I was challenged by the intricacies of technique and I devised a new surgical procedure for cleaning blood in patients with non-functioning kidneys. Soon after, my interests broadened to include basic medical research and I obtained a Ph.D. in experimental medicine, presenting my contributions on transplant rejection at international symposia. All this time, I practiced as a urologist and because I practice under the government Medicare system in Canada, I see a great many patients, many more than my U.S. counterparts. It became obvious that urology was more than simply surgery or medicine. Living, complex human beings came to me because my specialty and no other was the one concerned with a wide variety of sensitive and often disturbing problems. I began to note and apply myself, not only to medicine and surgery, but to the other very real needs of my patients: for information, encouragement, and advice.

The vast majority of mankind, no matter how successful or intelligent, is surprisingly ignorant when it comes to bodily functions and disorders. I suspect the average man turns a blind eye to health matters—until a problem arises, and then he panics. I remember one patient, a world-renowned professor, suggesting that his abuse of chocolates was the cause of a newly discovered cancer. Another patient, a lawyer, asked me where his kidney might be. He had no idea whether the organ was in his chest, abdomen, or pelvis. A university professor asked me whether the carving out of his prostate gland would change the sound of his voice. A successful business-man wondered whether he could catch his wife's cervical cancer. I have seen men turn green and faint with just a gentle touch of their genitalia. "Anywhere else, Doc, but I just can't stand to be touched there." Educated, intelligent people become inconsistent and irrational when they have to deal with health problems of their private parts.

This book is the answer to all the questions I have ever been asked—timidly, angrily, curiously—in the sanctity of my office. Questions about why urination has become painful or difficult, if a vasectomy cuts potency, the pros and cons of circumcision. Questions about which partner is infertile, what treatments are available, and what exactly is artificial insemination. Taking care of these concerns is what I do every day. No question is irrelevant. I have been around long enough to know that private parts, although taboo, are of vital interest.

In this book, I will talk as if I were talking to a friend or a patient in my office. I will explain puberty, erection, orgasm, and the workings of the prostate in such a way that you can understand how your body functions. I will discuss the old and the new sexually transmitted diseases so that you can distinguish between media rumor and real risk. I will describe surgical procedures from the point of view of a surgeon and tell you how to choose a good doctor. Many of these questions and topics affect the vast majority of men at some time in their lives, yet are grossly misunderstood. I believe that understanding what's going on in your own body will help you. From what I have seen, knowing what can go wrong and what can be done about it makes things easier.

I pull no punches. This is a straightforward, honest effort. My goal is to eliminate traditional secrecy and make useful information easily available. If I can assuage the fears and help men deal realistically with the health of their private parts, I will have succeeded.

PRIVATE PARTS

1 PRIVATE PARTS: WHAT THEY ARE AND HOW THEY WORK

This book is about the male body; more precisely, about that part of the male body that can be covered by an athletic supporter. Many men refer to this part of the body as their "privates." The penis and the scrotum are on the outside, and the bladder, prostate, testicles, and other genital parts are inside the body. Often, men don't know very much about their privates—even, for example, where their prostate is located. To compound the problem, they are often too timid to ask questions. Reading this book will make you more informed and relaxed about this part of your body. It will give you a sense of what's normal, and what's not, what disorders can arise, and what can be done about them.

The first chapter begins with a simple description of where the various parts are located in the body, how they look, and how they function in a normal, healthy man. This basic overview will help orient you so that you can better understand the answers to your specific concerns as they are covered throughout the book.

THE PENIS This organ must be the focus of more male attention than all the *femmes fatales* in the world. I see countless patients who come to my office because they are preoccupied with the size and shape of their penis. "Shouldn't it be bigger?" "Do the bags hang right?" "I was hit by a baseball when I was ten years old, everything turned black and blue, that's why it's so small." I examine each one of these patients forthwith and, invariably, I see a perfectly normal organ.

1

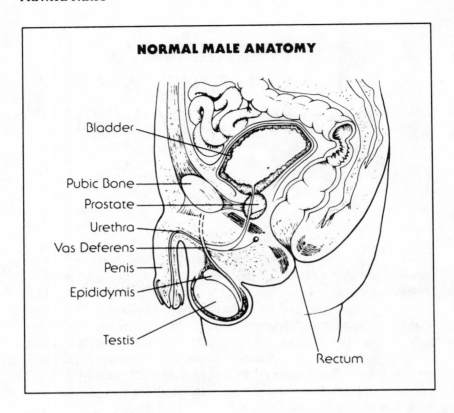

NORMAL MALE ANATOMY

Bladder

Pubic Bone

Prostate

Urethra

Vas Deferens

Penis

Epididymis

Testis

Rectum

If the preoccupation with penile size did not cause such real distress, it would be funny. Suffice it to say that the size of the penis has nothing to do with virility. Many men think women derive more pleasure from a larger penis but, in fact, a woman cannot tell the size of the penis from sensations in the vagina. Penis size is a male preoccupation. I have never heard a woman complain about the size of her partner's penis. Rigidity, or the strength of the erection, is more important to women and rigidity has nothing to do with size. Even men with a partial amputation of the penis, due to cancer, still have pleasurable intercourse.

As a ballpark figure, the average length of the flaccid penis is three to six inches, although some are shorter and some are longer. The length of the erect penis varies from four to eight inches, with the same proviso, and the average diameter at the base is about one and a half inches. Those who wish to hang on to a preoccupation with size may desist when they consider themselves as a species: the human penis, in relation to body size, is a paltry thing compared to other animals. The boar has a penis one and a half feet long; the stallion two and a half feet; the bull three feet; the elephant five feet; and the blue whale eight feet. . . .

The head of the penis, the glans, is covered by a sleeve of skin known as the foreskin. The amount of foreskin varies considerably and there is no problem for adults as long as the foreskin can glide easily over the head of the penis. The area under the foreskin should be cleansed daily with soap and water.

The shaft of the penis is covered by smooth hairless skin. Inside the shaft are three cylinders of erectile tissue: a pair on top, and a smaller cylinder below. This smaller cylinder contains the urethra and ends as a bulged head, which is the glans penis. The paired cylinders end just behind the glans and extend into the body, beyond the visible portion of the penis, to each side of the pelvic bone. The main nerve and the blood vessels run in the midline, on top, between the paired cylinders. Nerve tendrils branch out everywhere in the penis, but particularly to the head. Direct stimulation of these nerve endings produces man's most exquisite sexual sensations.

ERECTION The erectile tissue is in the three cylinders described above that make up the shaft of the penis. When the penis is in its flaccid state, the erectile tissue is like compressed dry sponge, with very little blood passing through: the blood that does flow into the penile artery is shunted directly into the outflow vein, bypassing the erectile tissue. When erection occurs, tiny trapdoors (named polsters) close off the shunt, and the erectile tissue fills with blood. This causes the penis to straighten out like a garden hose when a tap is turned on and the nozzle closed.

The polsters are activated in two ways. Sometimes, sexy thoughts send a message to the polsters via the sympathetic nerves. Other times, touching, rubbing, or other direct stimulation activates the polsters through the spinal column, like a knee jerk. Morning erections are often reflex erections, activated by the stimulation of a full bladder. If they occur in the absence of a full bladder, obviously other factors are at play. But whatever the cause, the presence of a morning erection means that, physiologically, all systems are go.

Of course, polsters are not actual physical structures. A search

3

for tiny muscles was undertaken at autopsy and came up with a blank. They are useful, however, as an explanatory concept. It is likely that chemical receptors are the polsters' physiological equivalent as, these days, it is possible to create an erection by injecting chemicals directly into the erectile tissue.

The erect penis assumes an angle of 140 to 160 degrees, give or take a few degress. This angle corresponds to the angle of the vagina. When the strength of erection is normal, but the angle is less than 90 degrees, it is possible to shorten the upper surface of the penis by surgically removing wedges from the coverings of the erectile cylinders. This is done so that intercourse can be comfortable.

INTERCOURSE Although intercourse is not the only form of sex play between consenting adults, it is often the ultimate act. The thrusting motions massage the penile nerve endings in a rhythmic manner to create a preorgasmic intensity which is almost always pleasurable.

Pain is uncommon and usually due to an injury of the tag of skin that runs from the foreskin to the undersurface of the head of the penis. If this tag tears and heals with a scar, erection and intercourse can pull on it to cause pain. A simple surgical repair, or a circumcision, cures the problem. Pain that is not due to this tag of skin, or to a disease process in the penis, is rare.

ORGASM When stimulation reaches a certain intensity, it triggers the waves of contractions we associate with orgasm: the bladder neck contracts; the muscles around the prostate gland, seminal vesicles, and vas deferens contract, squeezing juice into the urethral passage; the ejaculate forms a glob stretching the wall of the urethra and the muscles of the pelvis contract. The result is ejaculation and the pleasurable sensation of orgasm.

EJACULATION It is not uncommon for normal men to ejaculate two to five minutes after penetration. (Hours of thrusting and intricate swordplay seem more the stuff of novels than of daily life.) A man could be said to have premature ejaculation if he ejaculates before he penetrates the vagina, or if he ejaculates moments after penetration. Men who experience this problem frequently consult sexologists, who have a number of techniques to delay ejaculation. Some therapy involves mental training, and some involves physical reconditioning. In one particular technique, the head of the penis is pinched by either partner when ejaculation is imminent. This aborts the ejaculation. Intercourse is then resumed and the technique is practiced until a more satisfactory pattern of ejaculation is established. I have counseled a number of patients on this technique and many patients are helped by it.

Ejaculation is almost always pleasurable, creating, as it does, a sensation in the "pleasure center" of the brain. Painful ejaculation, however, is not an uncommon complaint. A number of middle-aged men complain that ejaculation sometimes hurts. I pay more attention to those who tell me it hurts all the time. In these cases, I check for cancer, or infection of the prostate gland. If the rectal examination of the prostate and the prostatic secretion are normal, I reassure the patient and suggest a heaping teaspoon of baking soda, four times a day, in a glass of water. Normal ejaculate is alkaline and I hope that by alkalinizing the body with baking soda, the symptoms will be alleviated. Although patients' reports are positive, I am not certain whether I am treating the symptom or the psyche.

The Ejaculate

The normal ejaculate varies in volume from one half a milliliter to eight milliliters give or take a milliliter, and the bulk of the fluid represents prostate secretions. Sperm represents only five percent of the total volume. This explains why men who have had a vasectomy don't see or feel any difference in their ejaculate.

Ejaculate fluid is milky, sticky, highly alkaline, and has a uniformly pungent odor. This odor is not due to the sperm as the ejaculate from a vasectomized man has the same odor.

A bloody or rust-colored ejaculate frightens most men. It may signify prostate cancer or infection, but most often it is as innocent as a nosebleed. Traditionally, men with a rusty ejaculate were treated with antibiotics, but recent studies have demonstrated that patients who don't take antibiotics do as well as those who do. I massage the prostate, produce a secretion, and treat patients only when the prostatic smear suggests a prostate infection or if the rectal examination suggests cancer.

5

THE URETHRA, PROSTATE, AND THE BLADDER

The urethra is a delicate, thin-walled tube, about eight inches long. It extends from its opening at the tip of the penis to the bladder.

In the penis, it is enveloped in spongy erectile tissue. Near the bladder, it is surrounded by the sphincter muscle, which keeps the urine in the bladder. Just beyond the sphincter, it is surrounded by the prostate gland and this is the site of possible prostate problems. Should the prostate enlarge, it is at this place that the urethra will be choked.

The urethral walls are made of unicellular "columnar" cells which lie one beside the other, like soldiers at attention. It is only at the head of the penis that the urethral lining changes to multilayered cells like those in the skin. Because the lining is so thin, catheters and instruments can easily poke through, causing scarring and blockage in the passage. This is why doctors think twice about medical intervention and this is also why it is so astounding to discover the assorted doodads men insert into their urethra.

Over the years, I have recovered a cornucopia of items from the urethra and the bladder. At different times, I have extracted a safety pin, a baby onion, a glass stirring rod, and a piece of stick, all deliberately inserted. The items have been inserted in an ill-conceived attempt to provide rigidity or, more often, in an attempt to enhance sexual pleasure. Since objects as soft and as pliable as a thin rubber catheter can irritate and damage the urethra, it should be stressed that under no circumstances should objects of any kind be inserted into this delicate passage.

The Prostate Gland

The normal prostate gland is about an inch and a half in diameter, an inch in length, and weighs about twenty grams. It is about as big as a chestnut or walnut.

Inside the prostate gland are glandular cells, muscle cells, and fibrous cells, intermixed with blood vessels, nerves, and surrounding fat. The glandular cells secret fluid that is important for sperm life, but the prostate has no vital function. Life can go on quite well without it.

In mid-life, this gland has a tendency to grow and choke off the flow of urine through the urethra. Yet it can enlarge to as much as two hundred grams without totally stopping the flow. Size alone is not a basis for surgery. The question really is: Does the man feel like urinating too often, day and night? Does he find his flow weak and uncomfortable? Does he have trouble knowing when his bladder has emptied? Discomfort can occur with a hundred-gram gland or a thirty-gram gland or, as in the case with half of all men over fifty, not at all.

The Bladder
The bladder is the balloon-like structure situated low in the abdomen just behind the pubic bone. When empty and collapsed, it is, in size and shape, like an uncooked egg out of its shell. When filled with urine, it resembles a grapefruit or a cantaloupe. The bladder fills with urine from the kidneys, transported by tubes called the ureters. A simple flap valve prevents the urine from flowing backward toward the kidney. As it fills, the walls of the bladder relax, accommodating the increased volume. At this point, no sensations are sent to the brain. When the urine volume reaches near-capacity, the bladder registers a sensation of fullness. When it is convenient, a message is consciously sent to the brain, the bladder muscles contract, the sphincter muscle opens, and the bladder empties.

If we try to make a bladder with synthetic materials, we run into enormous engineering problems. What is required is a receptacle, like a plastic bag, that can hold more and more fluid without changing the tension in its wall but which, near capacity, changes into a container with tension in its wall, so that it can contract and evacuate. It must have the features of a plastic bag when it is filling and metamorphose into a rubber balloon when full. Furthermore, the inner lining of the receptacle must not form encrustations despite the fact that microscopic crystals are present in the urine. The humble little bladder is a magnificent example of the intricacies of nature.

THE SCROTUM AND THE TESTICLES

The Scrotum
The scrotum is the skin bag that contains the testicles and their accessory structures. It is hairy and has a thin layer of muscle under the skin. When this muscle contracts, the scrotum shrinks and pulls the testicles closer to the body. When this muscle relaxes, the testicles drop away from the body. By regulating the distance of the testicles from the body, a

7

matter of inches, the temperature of the testicles remains four de-grees cooler than normal body temperature. The cooler temperature is important for healthy sperm production. Nylon-type bikini briefs pull the testicles toward the body and curtail sperm production. It is best to wear loose, cotton shorts.

The Testicles

Normal testicles can be as small as an egg yolk or as big as a large-sized plum. Large testicles do not mean more masculinity or greater fertility. Nor does the testicular size correspond to height or body weight.

Before birth, the testicles start life high in the back of the abdomen near the level of the kidney. They descend gradually and, by the eighth month in utero, are attached outside the bottom of the ab-dominal sac. In the final month before birth, they drop farther, into the bottom of the scrotum, pulling the bottom of the abdominal lining down with them. The piece of abdominal lining now in the scrotum is like the cellophane casing of a sausage closed at the bottom. In normal health, this tube of lining closes off at the top as well and is empty of the sausage. The potential opening is always present, however, and all men are susceptible to hernia formation, a condition in which the intestine is pushed into the tube.

Inside the testicle are a cluster of tubules separated by cells. The Leydig cells manufacture the male hormone, testosterone, and se-crete it directly into the bloodstream. The Sertoli cells nourish the tubular cells. The cells that line the tubules manufacture sperm. The transformation of a tubular cell into a sperm takes over seventy days—from the parent tubular cell, the spermatogonia, to the pri-mary spermatocyte, to the secondary spermatocyte, where the chro-mosome numbers are halved, to the spermatids, which develop tails to become the sperm. And this transformation is another scientific marvel.

THE ACCESSORIES   *Epididymis*

The epididymis is a comma-shaped structure that drapes over the back of the testicle, attached to it like a worm on a fruit. It is less than half an inch in width and just over an inch long. It has a head on top, a body in the middle, and a tail below.

8

When it is cut open, there is a cluster of tiny tubules inside. If the tubules are dissected out, the epididymis forms a continuous tube. Within the epididymis, the sperm mature and acquire the ability to swim. Sperm recovered from the head of the epididymis cannot swim and are unlikely to create a pregnancy, while those recovered from the tail are much more fertile.

Vas Deferens

The vas is continuous with the epididymis and conducts the sperm to its storage house, the seminal vesicle. The vas is about as thick as a wire coat hanger and is over a foot long. If it is cut open, the inside canal is hard to find as it is so small. The vas is almost all muscle, making it a hard cord easily felt through the scrotal skin. It takes the sperm on a long ride from the tail of the epididymis, up above the pubic bone, and back behind the bladder to join the seminal vesicle.

Seminal Vesicle

The seminal vesicle is an irregular-shaped structure about the size of a cigarette lying above the prostate, behind the bladder. It is connected to the vas in Y form so that a single duct, called the ejaculatory duct, drains both the vas and the seminal vesicles into the urethra. The seminal vesicle stores sperm. It also produces a sugar found in fruit, called fructose, which is found nowhere else in the body. In infertility testing, if the ejaculate contains no fructose, it means that the person was born without seminal vesicles and is irrevocably infertile. Theoretically, the seminal vesicles of one man can, in a lifetime, store all the sperm necessary to repopulate the world.

Since the groin and genital areas of the body have long been unmentioned and unmentionable in polite society, locker-room gossip and embellished anecdotes have too often been the source of information.

"Jimmy says that you can go bald playing with your pecker."

"How did he learn that?"

"Charlie told him that's how his uncle got bald."

Locker-room dialogue may be cute for teen films, but it is no help at all for learning to live with, and care for, your body. We all need real information for the changes and challenges of everyday life. This basic anatomy walk-through is only the beginning, and now we can go on to consider each of your specific concerns about every aspect of your private parts.

2 IMPOTENCE

My patient was a retired sixty-six-year-old man with the wrinkled, weathered complexion of a seasoned sailor.

"There are so many people here waiting to see you, and I'm not sick like them. I shouldn't be wasting your time. . . . It's just that my lady friend expects so much more," he began.

"You're not altogether dead down there, then," I replied, knowing that the reason for the referral was impotence.

"No, but it disappears on me so quickly, you see, before I can do anything."

"I understand."

"To be honest, I shouldn't be complaining. I've had my share in my lifetime, more than my share in my youth, I suspect. I can live with the memory. But it's kind of hard on my lady friend, you see. She does everything possible to help me, bless her. She rubs me, licks me, sucks me, anything to get it up. Her secret powder works some, but I was hoping that you doctors might have something more to offer."

"Secret powder?" I asked. "Is it something you mix in a drink?"

"No, no! You sprinkle it on. It prickles and burns a bit, but as I said, it helps."

"I've never heard of the preparation," I confessed.

"No kidding? Would you like to see it?"

"You have it with you?"

He said not another word but dug deep into his trouser pocket and extracted a worn envelope held together by a rubber band. He removed the rubber band and unfolded the envelope carefully. I felt

11

party to a conspiracy. He might have been showing me contraband opium or hot jewelry. I was spellbound. He pushed the envelope in my direction.

"May I see it?" I asked, my hand already extended.

He passed it to me, still silent, triumphant.

The powder was coarse, lemon-tinted, and speckled with dark green flakes. I examined it closely, then brought it to my nose. There was an odor I recognized immediately. I suppressed a smile but could hardly contain myself.

"Well, if it helps, I wouldn't knock it," I said, and passed him back the powdered chicken stock, the parsley flakes still clearly evident. . . .

I checked my patient thoroughly and ordered a series of tests. He was not on any medication associated with impotence, he had normal sensation in the genital area, and his blood hormone levels were normal. But tests showed poor circulation to the penis, indicating a physical basis for this man's impotence. Yet he had responded, somewhat, to the "secret powder," demonstrating, even in this case, the power of the psyche.

Traditionally, most impotence (as much as ninety percent) is considered to be of psychological origin—often attributed to the high levels of distress in our society. Many men live competitive and stressful lives. They are often driven by material success and by images of sexual prowess. Unrealistic expectations are fueled by a barrage of sexual innuendo—on billboards, in magazine ads, and on television commercials. Success is often equated with money and sexual performance. It is not surprising that the prototype of an impotent patient is the highly successful business executive—driven beyond the bounds of comfortable behavior into impotence. In fact, it is a common observation that ninety percent of the chief executive officers of the major corporations suffer from impotence.

Sometimes an individual confides that he is potent with one partner but not with another. In such a case, psychological factors are at play. And even if the case is not as clear cut as amorous preference, the task is often to discern and neutralize the upsetting psychological disturbances.

Psychiatrists keep busy with suicidal, depressed, and schizophrenic patients. Urologists are busy with surgical corrections. Thus impotence and other psychosexual problems, such as premature ejaculation and inability to ejaculate inside the vagina, have become the domain of sexologists. Unlike psychiatrists and urologists, sexologists need not be medical graduates. They are usually clinical psychologists with a master's degree who have chosen to concentrate on sexual problems.

Sexology is a relatively new discipline: its basic therapeutic principle, discovered and promoted by Masters and Johnson, is called sensate focusing. It involves the patient and his partner in a program of gradual progressions beginning with nongenital touching. The couple is encouraged to focus on general rather than genital sensation, deliberately delaying activities that might promote performance anxiety. Gradually, they progress to mutual masturbation and, finally, to intercourse. In the undiluted Masters and Johnson treatment, both partners, regardless of the perceived problem, undergo an intensive two weeks of therapy with the help of both a male and a female sexologist. But in many cities this full therapy is not available. Most sexologists work alone, with weekly appointments at best. Often the patient is alone. The sexologist may use erotic literature, videotapes, and techniques of direct counseling as well. Sexologists to whom I have referred patients tell me that when the patient is strongly motivated to recover his potency, has a cooperative partner, and is willing to make a series of visits with his partner, the results are most often satisfactory. Since there is no legal body equivalent to the American Medical Association to monitor sexologists, it is important to be sure that the sexologist is a specialized psychologist, trained in a center such as the one pioneered by Masters and Johnson.

How do we know if impotence is due to psychological or physical disturbances? There are three main categories of physical disturbance—circulation based, hormone based, and neurologically based—and it is necessary to consider these possible causes of impotence before deciding that the problem is psychological.

THE SCIENCE   *Impotence from Impaired Blood Flow*
                One of the first potential causes of physical impotence that I check for is the blood flow to the penis. Sometimes the small vessel that carries the main blood flow is blocked by a blood clot or plaque from hardening of the arteries. If this is the case, there is no danger that gangrene will occur as it would in the leg, nor infarct (death of tissue from lack of blood) as would occur in

13

the heart, lung, kidney, or brain. There is enough blood flow to keep the penis alive, but not enough to create an erection.

The man affected by this usually experiences total impotence with loss of morning erection, but no loss of libido (sexual desire). Often, he also has circulatory problems in other areas of the body, such as previous heart attacks, strokes, high blood pressure, diabetes, or elevated blood cholesterol.

The test used to pin down the diagnosis of a circulation-based impotence is the Doppler flow study. In this test, ultrasound waves are bounced off red blood cells as they flow through the artery. (The ultrasound detects red blood cells in the same way sonar detects objects underwater.) Different patterns are recorded according to the density of the red blood cells. The ultrasound pattern obtained from the penis is compared to the pattern derived from the leg or the arm. If there are significantly fewer red blood cells in the sound pattern from the penis, the patient has an impaired blood flow.

Another way to map circulation is to inject dye directly into the artery. This is called an angiogram, and is the way circulation to the heart is tested before a coronary bypass operation. It is also the way the blood flow to the leg is tested before a blocked artery in the leg is replaced by synthetic tubing. The dye which is injected into the artery is a colorless fluid that shows up like bone on an X ray. But this angiogram kind of "mapping" of the circulation is not normally done on the penis: the problem is that the dye needle might dislodge plaque from the arterial wall and further block the blood flow. Therefore we only do angiograms on young men if they have no heart disease and if their problem is an injury that might have damaged the artery to the penis. These are the candidates who can be helped by microsurgery, and so we do an angiogram to pinpoint the blockage. If the angiogram finds a blocked artery, it can be corrected using techniques like those used for coronary bypasses. (In coronary bypass surgery, a vein is taken from the leg. It is sewn at one end into a hole made in the healthy part of the artery, then extended beyond the blockage and sewn, at the other end, into the heart vessel. The vein thus bridges the blockage.) When the penis has to be revascularized, the technical challenge is much greater as the artery is considerably smaller. A small artery which extends from the groin to the abdomen and is not essential to normal functioning is taken down from the abdomen and sewn into the penile artery, thereby increasing the blood flow. The vessels are so small that they can be joined only by working under the microscope, and that is why this procedure is called microsurgery.

Another surgical technique that is being explored to correct circulation-based impotence ties off some of the veins that take the blood out of the penis so that more blood will remain within it. Dr. Ronald Virag of France pioneered this approach; others who have tried the technique have reported varying success.

Impotence Due to Hormone Deficiency
Hormones are chemicals released directly into the circulatory system. They affect our physical and psychological state. When the level of the male hormone, testosterone, is abnormally low, there is often a loss of sex drive and the onset of impotence. Although this is largely true, it cannot be assumed that the loss of libido is due to hormone deficiency, or that depressed hormone levels will always be associated with loss of libido. I have seen men with zero-level testosterone after having had their testicles surgically removed to control prostate cancer. Yet their libidos and potency were intact. Eventually these men will become impotent, but how they could be potent with zero-level testosterone is inexplicable.

The bulk of the hormone, testosterone, is made in the testicles, while a minute amount is made by the adrenal gland. The testicle need not be large and firm to be a healthy hormone producer. Tiny, shriveled-up testicles, perhaps useless as sperm producers, may be quite adequate as hormone producers.

It is not clear when and why the testicles stop producing testosterone if they have not been damaged or removed. There is no equivalent of the female menopause in men. Nevertheless, when testosterone is not being produced it can simply be replaced with periodic injections. Two hundred milligrams of a testosterone, such as Delatestryl, given intramuscularly every two to four weeks assures normal male sexual potential.

Impotence Due to Nerve Damage
Diabetes and specific nerve diseases of the genital area can produce neurological disorders which affect potency. When impotence is neurologically based it is likely to be associated with other symptoms. The bladder, or the bowel, may not work well. There is likely

15

to be a loss of sensation in the genital area. The anal sphincter is likely to be lax. And the reflex called the bulbocavernosus reflex—which causes the anal sphincter to contract when the head of the penis or clitoris is squeezed—is likely to be lost.

Whenever there is impotence due to nerve disease there are other symptoms as well. Impotence is always part of a systemic nerve damage. But major systemic nerve disease can exist without impotence. It is fascinating, for example, that a man who is paralyzed below the waist, a paraplegic, is not necessarily impotent. His erection, however, is produced exclusively by the mind since he can't feel sensation in the penis. And yet he is able to have an erection, experience orgasm, ejaculate, and become a father. This is because the nerve connection from the penis to the spinal cord is intact, even though the connection from the brain to the spinal cord is severed. Impotence due to nerve damage occurs when the nerve connection from the penis to the spinal cord is damaged.

Impotence Related to Drugs
Drugs for the treatment of high blood pressure, drugs to counteract psychiatric disorders, and drugs to counteract anxiety disorders often cause impotence. So do nicotine and alcohol. Nicotine constricts small blood vessels and alcohol depresses all sensation, including sexual sensation. Any person who can associate the beginnings of impotence with starting a new medication should discuss the problem with his doctor. It would be unwise to simply stop taking the medication, but it may be possible to substitute another drug.

If you are taking certain medications but have no problems with erections, it might be wise to skip the following four headings on drugs. What I do there is discuss the drugs associated with impotence. If you have erection problems associated with a new medication it may be helpful to look through the list. I have identified the drugs by their generic names followed by their trade names in parentheses.

Drugs to Treat High Blood Pressure Five percent of patients taking hydrochlorothiazide (HydroDIURIL, Esidrix), ethacrynic acid (Edecrin), or furosemide (Lasix) report impotence; just over twenty percent of patients on spironolactone (Aldactone) report decreased desire and impotence; impotence with methyldopa (Aldomet) is dose re-

16

lated, ten to fifteen percent if the dosage is under 1 gram, twenty to twenty-five percent when the dosage is 1 to 1.5 grams, and fifty percent when the dosage is 2 grams a day; guanethidine (Ismelin) when taken at dosages of more than 25 milligrams per day causes retarded ejaculation in fifty to sixty percent of patients, sixty percent report decreased desire, and ten percent impotence; hydralazine (Apresoline) at dosages of more than 200 milligrams per day is associated with decreased desire and impotence in five to ten percent; propranolol (Inderal) in high dosage such as 160 milligrams per day is associated with impotence; clonidine (Catapres) causes decreased desire and impotence in ten to twenty percent.

Drugs to Treat Psychiatric Disorders   Among the drugs used in psychiatric disorders, haloperidol (Haldol) causes impotence in ten to twenty percent; monoamine oxidase inhibitors (Nardil, Parnate) cause impotence in ten to fifteen percent and delay ejaculation in twenty-five to thirty percent; tricylic antidepressants such as imipramine (Tofranil) and amitriptyline (Elavil) cause impotence in five percent; lithium carbonate (Lithane) is associated with impotence in a small percentage of patients.

Antianxiety Pills   Antianxiety pills such as diazepam (Valium) and similar drugs can increase or decrease desire and can cause impotence, especially when taken in high dosages.

Miscellaneous Drugs   A decrease in sexuality has also been reported with a number of other medications such as cimetidine (Tagamet) used for stomach ulcers; clofibrate (Atromid-S), a drug used to treat high cholesterol levels; digitalis (Lanoxin), essential for treating heart failure; antihistamines (Benadryl, Chlortrimetan) used for hay fever and other allergic conditions; and anticholinergics (Pro-Banthine) used to treat an overly active bowel or bladder.

THE REMEDIES   I treat patients referred to me with impotence no differently than I do all my other patients. I take the history and carry out a physical examination. By the time I have finished the examination, I will have decided whether the impotence is psychological, physical, or a combination of both. These judgment calls are not iron-clad and are verified by a series of tests.

If I judge that the patient has impotence of a psychological origin,

I send him to the sexologist. The others have blood drawn to measure testosterone and blood sugar and are sent for the Doppler flow study. Before the results come in, I prescribe Yohimbine (a preparation made from the inner bark of an African tree) tablets, eight milligrams (four tablets) per day, increased to sixteen milligrams per day. I tell the patients the pills are not hormones, nor placebos; that they are safe, and that they appear to help about one patient in three. I suggest that they stop the pills if there are any undesirable side effects, and that they should not expect results until they have reached the sixteen milligrams per day dosage. I also suggest that if the pills do not work, the patient might consider the papaverine-phentolamine injection treatment, which blocks the outflow of blood from the penis. This is a relatively new method of injecting drugs directly into the penis. Almost all the patients who are not helped by the Yohimbine pills opt for the injection treatment.

I choose a deliberately small test dose when a neurological cause of impotence is suspected, and a larger dose when a circulatory cause is likely. The preparation is injected directly into the mid-shaft of the penis, deep into the side wall, using a tiny tuberculin needle. The pain is minimal. Erection occurs in about ten minutes and lasts half an hour to two hours. The dosage is then adjusted up or down according to the results. Once the dose has been ascertained, the patient is then instructed to prepare the injections and to administer the drugs himself. Papaverine is sold as a two-milliliter vial, containing sixty-five milligrams of the drug, and phentolamine comes as a five-milligram powder. The powder is reconstituted in sterile water. One sixth of each drug package is administered as the initial dose. I use the two drugs when cost is not a problem. The cost of papaverine is one tenth that of phentolamine. Papaverine is less satisfactory as the erection is not as strong.

I have used the injection treatment to treat impotence associated with diabetes, to treat psychological impotence, and to treat nerve-related impotence after removal of a cancerous bladder or prostate. The treatments are highly successful, although the dose requirements are quite varied.

The injection treatment does not work in all patients, nor do all patients find the injections acceptable. At this point, some patients will decline further treatment. Others are anxious to try the penile implant.

18

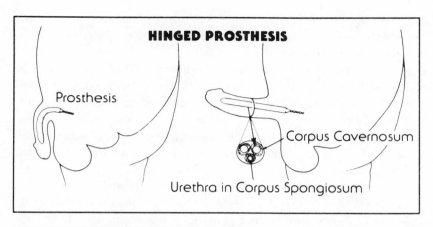

HINGED PROSTHESIS

Prosthesis

Corpus Cavernosum

Urethra in Corpus Spongiosum

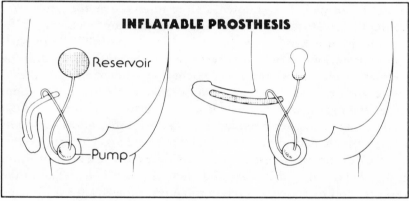

INFLATABLE PROSTHESIS

Reservoir

Pump

IMPLANTS An impotent man who has tried everything and is still impotent may consider a penile prosthesis. The idea of placing a rigid splint inside the body of the penis to counteract flaccidity may not seem so outrageous if you consider the whale or dog, both born with a bone in their penis. However, early attempts to splint the human penis with rib bone were not very successful since the bone tended to erode through the penis and break the skin.

Penile prostheses became a practical solution with the development of silastic—a material that combines silicon and rubber. Silastic is so inert that the body does not form scar tissue around it.

(Scar tissue would be the normal reaction to foreign matter in the penis.) Its tight network of fibrous cells, like the tendon of a muscle, creates a rigid nonpliable lump. Silastic avoids the scar tissue problem and makes the penile prosthesis possible. The first prosthesis, called the Small-Carrion prosthesis (after the doctors who developed it in 1973), was a rigid rod that filled two of the three compartments that make up the erectile body of the penis. It was immensely successful from day one, but the permanently erect penis was difficult to conceal. However, most patients simply strapped the penis to the abdomen and coped quite well.

Newer generations of prostheses have now flooded the market. I prefer the Finney flexi-rod with which I have had the most experience. This rigid silicone and rubber prosthesis has a soft spot built in it so that it normally hangs down. Before intercourse, the penis containing the prosthesis is lifted up by either partner to a comfortable entry angle. It is kept up by the vaginal walls and fulfills both partners' expectations of rigidity. There are prostheses that have flexible silver wires built in so they can be bent up or down, and prostheses whose girth and length I can custom-make in the operating room by peeling off the outer silastic layers or cutting off an end.

There are also several models of prostheses that allow the penis to be normally flaccid but that can be pumped up. The soft, hollow chamber of the prosthesis connects by tubes to a reservoir of water surgically placed in the lower abdomen. A pump is installed in the scrotum, and by squeezing the pump a few times, water is directed into the prosthesis. A release valve restores the flaccid state. The system is not fool-proof: tubes can leak, cylinders can fill up unevenly, and valves can fail.

The latest versions of the prosthesis with pump are self-contained units. By pressing the prosthesis in one spot, fluid is directed from one chamber to another, creating rigidity or flaccidity. Under the strain of sexual acrobatics, the apparatus has been known to collapse.

Slicker models will continue to challenge the market, but the price is skyrocketing. The self-contained pump models, for example, cost about $3,000.

I have inserted over a hundred prostheses of all varieties, and only once have I had a request to have one removed. The patient had become a widower and was certain that he had no further use for the prosthesis.

Men who have had their potency restored by the prosthesis experience pleasure and experience orgasm with ejaculation. The prosthesis, in other words, is not simply an apparatus to ensure the partner's satisfaction, or to restore a bruised male ego. Some patients have fathered children. In rare instances, if a degree of potency was present before, it may augment what is provided by the prosthesis. Patient satisfaction has been almost universal.

The Implant Operation
The penile prosthesis can be inserted in less than an hour, and the procedure is considered a relatively minor operation. In some hospitals, the operation is done on an outpatient basis, but I prefer to admit my patients.

I have used different skin incisions (a cut at the base of the penis, a circumcision cut, or an incision behind the scrotum), but a one-inch cut in the midline, at the point where the penis meets the scrotum, provides the easiest access. I cut the skin, then clear away the fat to expose the thick lining of the erectile tissue (*corpora cavernosa*). I incise the lining of the erectile tissue and easily insert a metal dilator into the spongy tissue. Then I slip in a prosthesis of the right length and close the opening like any other incision. The only departure from routine operative procedure is the use of copious amounts of antibiotic solution to wash the inside of the erectile tissue of the penis, and the incision itself, in order to reduce the risk of infection. A catheter that is normally inserted at the beginning of the operation is left in overnight. The pain and discomfort following the operation vary considerably from patient to patient, but pain-killing pills are usually necessary for two to eight weeks. Once the patient is pain-free, there will be no further discomfort. Intercourse can be attempted at any time after two weeks, but most patients are not ready for such activity for approximately eight weeks. My patients are normally hospitalized from one to three days.

In the early years of this operation, I could count on a number of visits from curious colleagues while performing the operation. I remember a visiting woman anesthesiologist remarking: "You never know when my husband may need one of these things!" Now the procedure has become so routine that there is no longer a flow of visitors.

SEX SHOP ITEMS   As far as sexual aids sold in sex shops or by mail-order houses are concerned, it is fairly well established that ginseng, Spanish fly, vitamin E, zinc, and multivitamin preparations are of little benefit in restoring potency.

"Cock rings" and suction devices, however, may help certain individuals. A "cock ring" is like a tourniquet applied to the base of the penis to retain a fleeting erection. It is slipped on after an erection has been achieved and it holds the blood in the penis to keep it erect. There can be problems if the ring is left on too long. One-half hour is considered an appropriate length of time.

For men who cannot achieve an erection at all, suction devices can help. In one model, for example, the penis is loaded into a suction apparatus. The vacuum sucks blood into the penis and is held there by a band like the cock ring. Recently I have begun prescribing the Osbon Erect Aid and I have been impressed with its efficacy even in those patients who were not helped by the papaverine-phentolamine injection. In another model, an apparatus that looks like a thick condom is fitted over the penis and mouth suction is applied to a small tubing that is attached to the "condom," which is left on during intercourse. If both partners are satisfied with these devices, there can be little harm in using them.

QUESTIONS AND ANSWERS   **What do I do if I can get an erection but it doesn't last?**

In younger men, this problem is almost always psychological and a sex therapist can be very helpful. In older men, this is not an uncommon problem. Some experts feel that excess venous drainage is the main problem and recommend surgically tying off some of the veins in the penis. The procedure can be successful, but not in all instances. A number of men have discovered that they can prevent a premature loss of erection by choking the base of their penis with a rubber band. I do not advise this, but a "cock ring" (sold at sex shops) may work.

Drug injections into the body of the penis will likely become the treatment of choice because they work.

Do injections into the penis work regardless of the cause of the impotence?

I have used the injection treatment to treat impotence associated with diabetes, to treat psychological impotence, and to treat nerve-related impotence after removal of a cancerous bladder or prostate. The treatments are highly successful regardless of what caused the impotence.

Isn't the injection into the penis very painful and aren't there complications?

The shaft of the penis is not overly sensitive. A tiny needle is used and most patients are surprised at how painless the procedure can be. There is a risk of infection, but the chances are remote. Of greater concern is the risk of a scar forming within the penis at the injection sites, causing curvature on erections as described in Peyronie's disease in Chapter 3. However, there has not yet been such a case reported. Sustained erection, well beyond two to four hours, occurs from time to time (in one to five percent of patients). This has been called priapism, but it is different from that condition in that there is no pain. However, if left untreated, these cases do develop all the complications associated with priapism: loss of oxygenation and scarring of the spongy tissue. Thus sustained erections associated with drug injections are treated like cases of priapism. First, an antagonist drug is injected. This is adrenaline as a one-in-one-thousand solution. If flaccidity does not result, the compartment within the penis containing the erectile tissue is drained with a needle and washed out with a salt and heparin solution. In cases where the penis still does not relax, a surgical drainage procedure is carried out. In the one case of priapism that I assisted, the erection was painless and therefore treatment was not sought for six hours. The condition did not respond to drug injections and required a surgical drainage procedure.

Painless prolonged erection, infection, and scarring inside the penis are possible complications, but so far they are very rare consequences of injection treatment. The injection treatment has been done in large numbers only during the past few years. Late complications from repeated use of needles are possible but have yet to be seen.

I have no qualms about recommending injection treatments for impotence despite these potential problems.

How good are pills and hormone shots for impotence?

Yohimbine, a preparation made from the inner bark of an African tree, and originally touted as an aphrodisiac, is now being used to alleviate impotence. Yohimbine has an effect similar to phentolamine, which blocks the outflow of blood from within the blood vessels. It is, therefore, not surprising that it helps twenty to thirty percent of patients with mild impotence. The pill is sold as a two-milligram tablet, and the effective dosage is four to eight pills per day, taken indefinitely.

Some people have tried testosterone preparations taken by mouth. But these preparations have to be taken in very large dosages and can injure the liver. Testosterone may be appropriate when the patient's blood serum shows a low level of testosterone, but in this case, intramuscular injections make sense.

Impotence has also been helped by placebos (pills which contain no active chemical). The healing qualities are taken on faith and faith seems to work.

I'm diabetic. Is impotence normal for my condition?

Diabetes is the single most common disease associated with impotence. The exact reason is unknown. Diabetes has been related to premature aging. The blood vessels of diabetics are particularly susceptible to degenerative changes. Impotence in diabetics may be circulatory in origin, although this has not been established.

I treat impotent diabetic men with the papaverine-phentolamine injections first. If there is no success, or if the patient is not happy with the response, I suggest a penile prosthesis.

Should I consider a penile prosthesis for my impotence? Will I be doing it for my partner or for myself?

A man with a prosthesis has the same sensual sensations as he would with a natural erection. The operation does not disturb the nerves that carry sensation. Thus what is originally felt remains unaltered. Pleasurable orgasms can be expected by both partners.

24

Can a woman tell if a man has a prosthesis?
No woman can tell the difference from sensations originating within the vagina. A knowledgeable woman can feel the difference with her hands.

How do I decide between an inflatable or a noninflatable prosthesis?
Basically, it is a matter of cost. The self-contained inflatable prosthesis costs about $3,000 and the noninflatable variety costs less than $1,000. Cosmetically, the inflatable type is preferable because it is less prominent in one's underwear. Functionally, there is no difference.

How soon after having surgery for a penile prosthesis can I have intercourse?
This depends on pain and discomfort, and these are somewhat variable. Most patients are not functional for about two months. After two weeks, there is little risk of damaging either the wound or the prosthesis, but most patients are reluctant to have intercourse until they are completely comfortable.

Can the prosthesis be removed?
Removal of the prosthesis is a very minor procedure, and can be done in the doctor's office. However, natural erection will not return because the erectile tissue will have been damaged.

3 THE PENIS

CIRCUMCISION **S**hould a newborn baby boy be circumcised? Parents whose religion offers them a choice will get mixed advice from the medical profession on this subject. The arguments advanced *against* the procedure might be as follows:

(a) The procedure constitutes unnecessary surgery with no medical or hygienic justification.

(b) The uncircumcised head retains more sexual sensitivity.

(c) The foreskin may prove useful as a source for skin grafting.

(d) An accident may occur with the procedure, leaving the infant mutilated.

(e) The American Academy of Pediatricians in 1971 and the American College of Obstetricians and Gynecologists in 1978 have declared circumcision medically unnecessary.

Doctors who *favor* circumcision at birth refute these arguments as follows:

(a) How can circumcision be considered unnecessary when cancer of the penis, phimosis (inability to retract the foreskin over the head), and paraphimosis (the foreskin gets retracted beyond the head and cannot be returned) can only occur in uncircumcised men?

(b) Foreskin protection of enhanced sensitivity may be faddish and overrated. Men who have undergone circumcision in adult life do not report noticeable differences in sexual enjoyment.

(c) The number of times foreskin skin grafts have played a significant role in the health of a patient is inconsequential.

(d) Mutilation of the penis at circumcision is a freak accident, like an amputation of the wrong limb. It can happen, but cannot be advanced as solid argument.

(e) Ask any man who has had to have a circumcision as an adult if he would not have preferred the procedure at birth. Ask the patient with cancer of the penis. Urologists, I suspect, favor circumcision on newborns. Seeing a case or two of cancer of the penis can affect one's outlook significantly.

Circumcision is a simple procedure and ritualistic circumcisions are done by mohels of the Jewish religion without formal surgical training. Newborn baby boys are often circumcised by pediatricians a few days after birth in a hospital by the "bell-clamp" method without an anesthetic. In the bell-clamp procedure an apparatus that looks like a thimble is put over the head of the penis, and the foreskin is pulled over it. A second part of the instrument then clamps down on the foreskin against the thimble and cuts off the foreskin. Every baby cries lustily throughout the ordeal, but I am not certain whether the infant is objecting to being strapped down or to the clamp.

When I was in training, I remember a senior urologist telling me that in a pinch any doctor can perform a circumcision. As specialists in the field, he suggested, we should be prepared to offer more. The procedure he recommended removes skin, but nothing more. If an analogy is made to a down-filled jacket, we can shorten the sleeve by slicing off the end such as in the bell-clamp method, or we can cut the outer material and the lining and push the filling up in the sleeve. By leaving behind the tissue between the outer and inner skins, we leave behind the vessels and nerves. There is less discomfort, less chance of bleeding, and an earlier return to normal functioning. One doctor on whom I carried out such a circumcision told me he was sexually functional in two weeks. It is a technique I have employed throughout my professional career.

ORNERY FORESKIN AND OTHER PROBLEMS

Tight Foreskin (Phimosis)

Phimosis is a condition in which the uncircumcised foreskin cannot easily be pulled back to a position behind the widest part of the head of the penis. The condition is associated with excess fore-

27

skin. It can also develop after an irritation has torn the skin and healing has contracted the foreskin.

The simple and only acceptable remedy is to carry out a circumcision. (It is possible to insert a forceps into the narrow foreskin opening and to stretch the channel open or to slit the foreskin vertically on top, but these are inferior methods of treatment since they run the risks of recurrent problems.)

Trapped Foreskin (Paraphimosis)
A paraphimosis occurs when a tight, uncircumcised foreskin is pulled back behind the head of the penis and cannot be returned. A tight ring is created above the head of the penis. The foreskin around the head swells up, just like a choked ring finger would, to the point where it is sometimes difficult to distinguish the head of the penis from the swelling. If the situation is not corrected rapidly, within hours, there is progressive swelling and an enormous collection of fluid will distort all normal anatomy: the trapped foreskin can accumulate so much fluid that the tip of the penis may appear to be five times its normal size. The solution is to squeeze all the fluid out of the area and to gently return the foreskin to its original position. When this is not possible, the skin is slit at its point of constriction in order to achieve repositioning. When the swelling has subsided, a formal circumcision is advised to prevent recurrences.

Paraphimosis commonly occurs with masturbation or bike-riding in children. In older men, the cause is often iatrogenic (doctor induced). For example, the foreskin may have been pulled back for catheterization and forgotten to be replaced.

Bent Penis (Peyronie's Disease)
More than two hundred years ago, a French doctor, François de la Peyronie (1743), described an affliction of the penis that has a dramatic manifestation: Nothing much is obvious when the penis is flaccid, but upon erection the penis will curve upward ten to thirty degrees, and sometimes ninety degrees and more. When the curvature is severe, there is pain on erection and intercourse becomes impossible. This strange condition is called Peyronie's disease.

In the years that have passed since the original description, we have learned some things about this disorder but nothing about its cause. No causative virus, bacteria, or chemical imbalance has been identified. What has come to light is the apparent statistical association of the condition with moderate alcohol intake, and its frequent statistical association with a scarring process in the hand called Dupuytren's contracture. Why the two conditions often occur together is not known. In Dupuytren's contracture, the tendons that allow the ring and little finger to close into a fist get pulled down by scar tissue, keeping the two fingers in a closed position. The tendons in the palm become prominent and obvious. A releasing procedure can be carried out by a plastic surgeon.

Peyronie's disease is scar tissue and nothing more. It affects the tough elastic lining of the penis's spongy erectile tissue. The scar forms on the lining and does not allow that part of the penis to expand during erection. So the penis curves around the lesion. Under the microscope nothing special is found in the scar. Like other scars anywhere in the body, however, calcification can occur, making the lump harder.

Patients who develop this malady naturally fear it might be cancerous since it is often felt as a hard lump. Peyronie's disease is not a cancer and never becomes a cancer. This reassurance can be offered with confidence. Predictions about what can happen are much less certain. The condition can improve spontaneously, stay the same, or worsen.

Over the years, a number of different treatment regimens have been recommended. These include vitamin E by mouth, a pill called Potaba (potassium para aminobenzoate), injections of cortisone directly into the hard area, and X-ray treatment. One study found that leaving the patient alone was as effective as any of these treatments. I offer vitamin E to my patients (two hundred milligrams three times a day) because I know that this will do no harm.

When erection becomes painful or intercourse impossible, surgical correction is considered. The operation devised by Dr. Charles Devine and Dr. Charles Horton of Eastern Virginia Medical School is quite successful. The scar is surgically removed and replaced with a graft of the inner skin layer, called the dermis, obtained from the thigh or lower abdomen. When the condition is very advanced, the dermal graft application is not very successful and the better solution is often the insertion of the penile prosthesis.

Painful, Undesired Erection (Priapism)

A state of sustained, unrelenting erection, usually associated with pain and unaccompanied by any sexual desire, is the symptom of a medical condition called priapism. It must have been a doctor with some schooling in Greek mythology who first named the condition after the Greek god of fertility—Priapus. Priapus had a huge phallus, and in this sense the label is appropriate. It seems inappropriate, however, to name the condition after a god of fertility because the end result of priapism is usually impotence and infertility.

Priapism occurs most often, for no apparent reason, in the sexually active male. The condition can also occur when the natural flow of blood in the penis is altered by injury, drugs, or blood disease such as sickle cell anemia or leukemia. When there is a known factor promoting the condition, the disease is called secondary priapism.

The critical problem in priapism is the venous drainage system. The blood wells up in the penis, cannot escape, loses its oxygen, and promotes clot formation, then scarring.

The diagnosis is often delayed because the patient is embarrassed and fails to seek medical attention right away. Sometimes, intercourse is attempted and found too painful, at which point medical advice is sought. As with most medical problems, the shorter the interval between the onset of symptoms and treatment, the better the results.

The first few hours are usually spent administering pain-killing drugs, ice-water enemas, and drugs to lower blood pressure. As a rule, if there were any doubts about the diagnosis, these doubts are quickly dissipated by the failure of the patient to respond. More aggressive measures are then instituted. The hard body of the penis is pierced with a large needle. If dark, almost black blood is recovered, the penile compartment is washed out with an anticoagulant saline solution until the return flow is pink, and proper venous drainage established by one of several techniques. Despite these valiant efforts, the risk of eventual impotence is substantial. So much so, in fact, that doctors treating this condition insist on covering themselves with explicit consent. It is a sad commentary on our society that physicians who administer emergency care during non-business hours can face litigation when the results are unsatisfactory to the patient. Still, I don't know a doctor who would not attempt to salvage a functional penis even when the condition is advanced and the successful recovery of potency is unlikely. On the other hand, if the priapism is not of long standing, the treatment is usually quite successful.

Cancer of the Penis

Men who have been circumcised at birth never develop cancer of the penis. (Boys who are circumcised in their youth rarely develop the cancer.) Cancer of the penis occurs virtually exclusively in men who have never been circumcised. In all probability the most vulnerable men are those who have not been circumcised and who have phimosis. It is suspected that a peculiar bacteria called the *smegma bacillus* promotes cancer formation. One Japanese investigator patiently and painstakingly painted the *smegma bacillus* on rabbit penises for years but failed to produce cancer. If it had worked, he would have pinned down the cause and effect relationship, although the fact that he didn't does not preclude the possibility. It only means that the *smegma bacillus* may not produce penile cancer in rabbits.

By pulling back the foreskin, uncircumcised men can detect a cancer right away. It is painless but first looks like a raised lump, then, as it grows, more cauliflower-like. Prompt attention at this point is almost always curative. When cancer is discovered early, treatment with anticancer drugs incorporated into a cream such as 5-fluorouracil cream might control the disease. Radiotherapy can also cure the disease in its early stages. When the cancer becomes invasive, or digs in its roots, it is necessary to amputate a portion of the penis.

This is accomplished at a point one inch from the visible margin of the cancer. Usually, there is sufficient length left to allow a cosmetically acceptable result. The patient can still direct his urine stream and can resume his sex life. In my experience, patients who have lost the head and up to two thirds of the shaft of their penis report that they and their partners have resumed a normal sex life.

Sometimes, there is insufficient length to retain any portion of the visible penis because of an extensive cancer. Under these circumstances, the urine flow is diverted to exit behind the scrotum. (Patients will have to sit to void, but there will be voluntary control.)

When the cancer is confined to the penis, the results of surgery are quite satisfactory. Too often, the patient visits the doctor when the disease has already spread beyond the penis and into the lymph nodes, the glands that you can feel in the groin. A wider excision, with removal of lymph nodes, is sometimes carried out, but the results are less successful. Our hopes lie with better chemotherapy. Drugs which are presently available are not very effective for cancer of the penis, although the highly toxic anticancer drug called Bleomycin has been used with limited success.

It is always baffling to me when a patient comes in with such advanced disease. More than once I have seen a man of means, immaculately groomed, accompanied by a loving wife, pull back his uncircumcised foreskin and reveal an advanced cancer with its foul, dead tissue. Imagine a rotting cauliflower: that is what it is like— and the groin is filled with enormous matted nodes. How could it have been ignored to this degree?

Cancer of the Urethra

Cancer that originates in the urethra is exceedingly rare. In almost thirty years of treating patients with urological problems, I have seen no more than three or four patients with a cancer that started in the urethra. (Cancers that have spread to the urethra from original growths in the bladder or prostate are more common.) It is fortunate that this cancer is so rare because it is deadly. I have yet to see a patient survive it.

I remember one elderly woman in her late seventies. She could not empty her bladder, and on examination, no instrument would pass into her bladder because of a blockage in the urethra. The blockage was due to the cancer. We performed a major operation and cut out the urethra and bladder. She survived the operation, but the cancer recurred in other parts of her body and she did not live a year. I recall another patient who was in his early fifties. He had difficulty passing urine and, on examination, a lump could be felt inside the mid-shaft of his penis. I was a resident doctor at the time, and like the other residents we all thought he had shoved some foreign object into his urethra. We were all ashamed when we discovered the lump was a cancer, and heavy with guilt when he died a few months later.

Cancer of the urethra is deadly because in its early stages the disease does not show any symptoms. By the time symptoms such as bleeding or difficulty with urine flow occur, or when a lump can be felt, the cancer has usually spread beyond the urethra. Surgery cannot remove all the microscopic deposits of the cancer. Chemotherapy may help, but because the cancer is so rare, valid treatment protocols have not been developed.

Misplaced Opening
The urethra should end at the tip of the penis. Sometimes, in an otherwise well-formed penis, the urinary opening is on the shaft of the penis on top, a rare condition called epispadias. More commonly, the opening is on the undersurface and is called a hypospadias. When the opening is almost at the head, the anomaly need not be corrected as it does not interfere with urination or reproduction. When the opening is in the shaft portion of the penis, or where the penis joins the scrotum, it is often associated with a downward curvature of the penis. This makes normal urination difficult and intercourse impossible. A number of techniques have been devised to correct the disorder and, on the whole, the surgical results are satisfactory, both cosmetically and functionally. Success is most assured when the procedures are done on children by urologic surgeons who confine their practice to children.

Medical problems associated with the penis can be bizarre. By and large, however, the problems are routine, occasionally made more difficult by men's inhibition, stoicism, and reticence to talk about malfunctions of their sexual organs. It is always best to see a doctor as soon as you notice something uncomfortable or unusual, even if you are embarrassed. The doctor is used to medical problems of all kinds and his job is to keep you healthy. You can help him by being cooperative, consulting him at an early stage.

QUESTIONS AND ANSWERS

Would you have your son circumcised?
Yes. One simple procedure at birth circumvents a lifetime of possible problems. Apart from the fact that only uncircumcised men get cancer of the head of the penis, uncircumcised boys have four times as many health problems associated with the head of the penis as do circumcised boys. The two specialty groups that have taken a stand against routine circumcision, the pediatricians and the gynecologists, are not

the ones who do circumcisions on boys or adults. Nor do they treat men with inflammation of the head of the penis, with phimosis and paraphimosis, or men dying of penile cancer.

Does cancer of the penis occur in circumcised men?
A cancer of the pigment-producing skin cells, called melanoma, can start in the skin of the penis. However, cancers that start at the head occur only in uncircumcised men.

Does anybody survive advanced cancer of the penis or urethra?
Yes, when the lymph nodes are not involved. Even cases necessitating almost total amputation, in which patients have to sit to urinate, are cured when there is no lymphatic involvement. But in my practice, I have never seen a patient survive when the original presentation included involvement of the lymph nodes.

Do women get anything like cancer of the penis?
Cancer of the vulva is the female equivalent. Both cancer of the penis and cancer of the vulva originate in skin cells. Cancer of the vulva is more common than penile cancer.

When I'm erect, my penis curves up and I feel a hard lump. Do I have cancer?
If you have a history of curvature on erection and if the lump is in the middle of the curvature, you have Peyronie's disease. Cancer never appears this way.

My penis curves on erection and I'm worried about injury to my partner.
I have heard men with very severe curvature tell me that their partners feel no discomfort. I have also seen men with minimal curvature tell me that their partners complain of pain. I doubt that it is the curvature that is the cause of painful intercourse for the partner.

When do I have to worry that my erection is lasting too long?
A sustained erection is not abnormal unless the erection is painful and devoid of any desire. If it is painful, unwanted, and has exceeded four hours in duration, it is a condition called priapism. External

examination of the penis cannot distinguish between sustained erection and priapism. Priapism requires prompt medical attention.

Why does impotence occur after priapism?
Scar tissue inside the penis destroys the ability of the spongy erectile tissue to expand. When erectile tissue canot expand, erection cannot occur.

Can impotence because of priapism be treated?
The impotence can be treated by insertion of a penile prosthesis. No other forms of treatment will work.

4 THE PROSTATE GLAND

Almost every man will have prostate trouble sometime in his life. Most often, the trouble occurs after age fifty when fifty percent of the male population develops a gradual enlargement of the prostate gland that slowly chokes off the urine flow. The cause of benign prostate enlargement is unknown and, to date, there are no pills to shrink the gland. The disease is rare in Japanese men living in Japan, becomes more frequent in Japanese living in Hawaii, and is as common in Japanese-Americans as it is in the rest of the American population. Thus the traditional Japanese diet—low in fat and red meat, and high in fiber—probably curtails prostate enlargement, although no tests have been undertaken to prove this. Since eunuchs never develop prostate enlargement, there is, it seems, a causative link between testosterone and prostate enlargement. "Health" food stores promote pumpkin seeds and other "natural" products as a cure, but if such simple products were an effective remedy, the pharmaceutical industry would have synthesized the active ingredient long ago.

Not as many men over fifty develop prostate cancer as develop prostate enlargement, although it is the third most common killing cancer in man. In men under fifty, the gland commonly becomes infected with microorganisms which reach the gland from the bloodstream or from the urine. Unlike infections in most other organs, prostate infection is exceedingly difficult to eradicate.

Given these realities, it makes sense that an appreciation and understanding of this gland and how to care for it should rate as a high priority for every thinking adult male.

ENLARGEMENT   *Symptoms*

When prostate enlargement begins to choke the urine flow, there will be a combination of a number of symptoms. These symptoms are:

1. Slow start
2. Weak flow
3. Dribbling at the end
4. Need to go often
5. Need to get up often at night

The symptoms develop so insidiously that older men accept the disability as part of the aging process. A slow start, particularly in the morning, is usually the very first symptom. By itself, it is not a cause for alarm. There are many men who can never void in public nor on command. They need privacy and there is nothing wrong with that.

A weak flow is one of the symptoms of prostate trouble. Often the stream is slow and stops and starts on its own accord. Slow streams and an interrupted flow mean blockage. This may be acceptable to one person and may not be acceptable to another so that one man may choose to have a prostate operation and another may simply live with the discomfort.

Dribbling at the end of the flow is perhaps the most annoying symptom of an enlarged prostate. The flow trickles to a dribble which goes on endlessly. Imagine leaving the toilet only to find more drops coming through to wet one's underwear.

The need to go often during the day and night can be reasonably explained. The bladder is not being emptied completely at urination. This can be documented by X ray. The enlarged prostate can also cause irritation of the sensitive neck area of the bladder. This can trigger a desire to empty. Finally, the poor flow and lack of complete emptying promotes urinary infection that can stimulate frequent urination.

If the symptoms are ignored, the story can evolve in one of two directions. There can be progressive pressure damage to the urinary tract, eventually causing kidney damage. This is most uncommon today. The more likely result is acute and total inability to pass urine. This urinary retention may be precipitated by a drinking binge, a car trip when the call of nature could not readily be accommodated, or some kind of illness or surgery. The agony of urinary retention

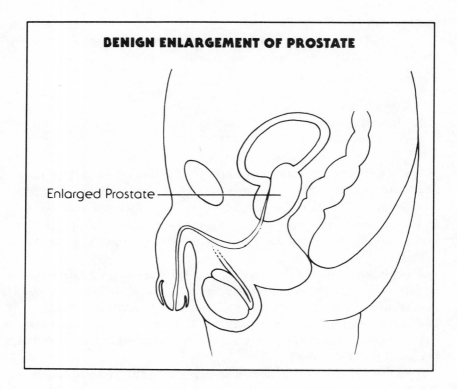

DENIGN ENLARGEMENT OF PROSTATE

Enlarged Prostate

has few parallels, and its relief by catheter insertion is consummate relief, as anyone who has been through the experience will testify.

Let me correct one pervasive misconception. There is no direct correlation between gland size as detected by digital rectal examination and degree of urinary symptoms. A doctor can render a disservice to a patient by expressing alarm at the size of the prostate when there are no complaints about urine flow. The size of the gland, per se, is never an indication to proceed with surgery. Intervention for the benign disease should be considered only when the symptoms become sufficiently bothersome.

What to Do
The solution to bothersome prostate enlargement is surgery. If the patient is well, with no other medical problems of consequence, he

just needs his plumbing fixed. The routine care will vary depending on the doctor and hospital.

My routine is as follows:

Pre-Op Tests

I like to make sure the kidneys are free of disease by using ultrasound examination or X ray. A clear fluid that contains a chemical with iodine is injected into a vein in the arm. Since arteriosclerosis does not occur in veins, there is no danger that the needle will release plaques, as it might in an artery. The injection, therefore, is safe and the chemical is quickly eliminated by the kidney. An X-ray picture taken at intervals shows up the chemical in the same way it shows bone, outlining, in sequence, the substance of the kidney and the urine in the kidney, ureter, and bladder. A film taken after emptying the bladder shows the amount of urine left behind. This series of kidney X rays is called the intravenous pyelogram (IVP). It is the single most useful X-ray test of the urinary tract. It cannot be used in people who are or may be allergic to iodine. There is a one-in-ten-thousand chance of a fatal allergic reaction. In practice not much attention is paid to this risk because it is so rare. The test is ordered with caution in people who are diabetic, or who have damaged kidney function.

The ultrasound alternative is totally safe. Sound waves that we cannot hear are bounced off different organs of the body. The pictures that are produced look like a radar screen in action. An ultrasound expert can decipher these bewildering pictures with amazing accuracy. What I get are still photos of the radar movie and the ultrasonographer's report, which I use to guide my diagnosis.

I check the anatomy near the prostate by direct inspection with an instrument called the cystoscope. This instrument is like a miniature periscope. The eyepiece is like that of a binocular; the shaft is about a foot and a half long and has the diameter of a pencil. The instrument is inserted directly into the urinary passage that has been lubricated and frozen with a local anesthetic. The fiber-optic light source and microlens system allows very accurate examination. There may be some discomfort, but there should be no real pain associated with the examination. Of course, the degree of discomfort will depend on the individual anatomy, any disorder, and the skill of the surgeon. The cystoscopic examination will clarify the degree of prostate enlargement and whether the right surgical approach is through the urinary passage. Sometimes, I combine the diagnostic examination (cystoscopy) with the prostate operation. Without the cystoscopy, the patient is saved an unpleasant test, but there is a risk of a surprise finding at surgery—like finding a scar in the passage (stricture of the urethra) or a bladder tumor. As a rule, prostate surgery can be better planned with a separate cystoscopy done beforehand.

Before the patient is admitted to the hospital, he has more tests. These include:

1. chest X ray
2. electrocardiogram
3. complete blood count
4. serum chemistry

These tests are routinely undertaken because the patient's account of his illness and the physical examination may not have uncovered problems that would be hazardous with prostate surgery. For example, the chest X ray may reveal tuberculosis or lung cancer. The electrocardiogram may show a silent heart attack, or an irregular beat. The blood count may indicate anemia or leukemia. In some cases, the blood chemistry is out of line: the potassium may be low, the calcium may be high, or the blood sugar may be sky high. When these preoperative tests are normal, the patient is admitted to the hospital the afternoon or evening before surgery.

As I practice in a university hospital, an intern or resident will visit, retake the patient's story, and redo the physical examination —listening to the chest, palpating the abdomen, and perhaps performing a rectal. There are pros and cons associated with being in a teaching hospital. Some of my patients are annoyed that they have to submit to an examination by a young doctor in training. And yet some of these same patients are most grateful that a resident doctor was immediately available in their moment of distress. The resident staff is also a final check on the propriety of the operation proposed. (I have, on occasion, changed my management of a case because of a new insight provided by my resident.) Personally, if I ever needed hospital care, I would choose a teaching hospital because of the continual presence of the residents. Odds are, a doctor would be at your bedside faster in a teaching hospital than in a nonteaching hospital.

In the afternoon of the day before surgery, an anesthesiologist will visit the patient. He or she will suggest the appropriate anesthetic— a general or a spinal. The patient may have a preference because of a bad experience with one or the other, or the anesthesiologist may indicate a preference for a particular patient. Generals are preferred if a previous back operation complicates the chances of getting the needle into the spinal column, or with heart disease, since, with a general, the anesthesiologist feels he can better control the administration of different drugs. In most cases, however, the spinal anesthetic is preferred for the procedure because there are fewer lung complications.

The Surgery
Let me describe exactly what is involved in prostate surgery done through the penis. After the administration of the anesthetic, the legs are placed in padded stirrups in a position like that of a woman delivering a baby. The genitalia are then washed with detergent and water. Sterile drapes cover everything except the penis. The urethra is then lubricated, measured, and a surgical instrument called the resectoscope is introduced. The resectoscope is similar to the cystoscope but contains an electrically heated wire loop for cutting. The loop is electrically activated by a foot pedal, and moved back and forth by finger control. The obstructing prostate tissue choking the urethra is carved out in little pieces the size of earthworms. When spurting blood vessels are encountered, a second foot pedal changes the electrical current and that cauterizes the bleeding vessel. It takes about an hour to complete the procedure, and the bits of cut tissue are flushed out with water through the hollow tube of the resectoscope. But the prostate tissue often remakes itself after each bite of the resectoscope much like shifting sand fills in a hole. So the craftsmanship required is not unlike that of a sculptor. At the completion of the procedure the inside of the prostate is a carved-out cavity.

Now a soft hollow tube, called a Foley catheter, which has an inflow tract and an outflow tract, is passed into the bladder. A continuous saltwater irrigation of the system is carried out for a day or

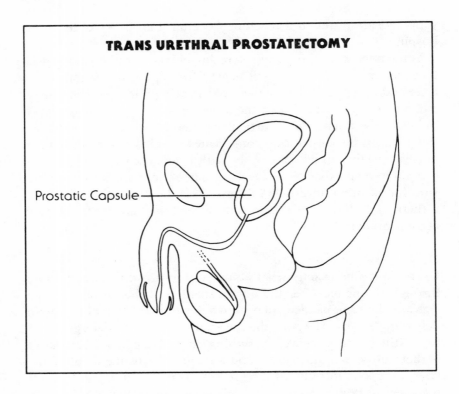

TRANS URETHRAL PROSTATECTOMY

Prostatic Capsule

two. Prostate surgery done in the manner described, through the natural channel and called transurethral prostatic resection (TURP), is the most common operation done for the benign enlargement. It is the least taxing and least stressful method for the patient. It has not always been so. Transurethral prostatic resection was long considered one of the most difficult operations for the surgeon to learn. And it was often a bloody mess.

The development of the fiber-optic light source and microlens system revolutionized this operation. Fiber-optic light allows powerful light beams to be transmitted along innumerable glass fibers made into a cord. The cord can be twisted and bent. The microlens system has upgraded the optics from a baby Brownie to a Nikon. Thirty years ago, the battery light source and the lens were such that when there was bleeding from one major vessel the procedure often had to be terminated.

The operating time for this procedure should be under one hour, although an hour and a half is not uncommon nor necessarily harmful. When the operation takes longer, there is an increased risk of injury to the passage (urethra) with potential formation of a scar or stricture. For the vast majority of patients the operation takes one hour, and the catheter can come out after one or two days. After the catheter is removed, there may be considerable amounts of blood mixed with urine in the initial period, but the flow should be better almost immediately. The patient usually leaves the hospital after four or five days.

Complications
Lung complications such as pneumonia or fluid in the lung are frequent in high-risk cases. Patients who are vulnerable include smokers, elderly men over seventy years of age, men who are more than a hundred pounds overweight, and men with known lung diseases. Smokers have two to six times the lung complications of nonsmokers. If smokers quit three months before surgery, they better their odds.

Convalescence
During the period of convalescence that follows, most patients tire easily and they must learn to give in to that. The reason for the fatigue is that there has been moderate blood loss during and after the operation. This blood is mixed with the urine and eliminated normally. There is also a risk of brisk blood loss up to the end of about five weeks and it's best not to stray too far from town until the risk period is over.

Lovemaking can be resumed in two months. However, ejaculation will be dry after prostate surgery: the ejaculate is being discharged into the bladder. It does no harm and is eliminated mixed with urine. But the sensation of orgasm is not lost. On the other hand, approximately thirty percent of patients report varying degrees of impotence following prostate surgery. Some men are unequivocal about the loss of potency. The usual explanation for this has been that the procedure is being carried out on older men who normally take longer to achieve erection. And men may prefer to attribute the loss of potency to a particular event in their lives rather than accept a progressive change in sexual prowess. But the majority do not suffer any loss of potency.

The patient can be home in under one week, and convalescence lasts one month. Indeed, patients have little control of all but the convalescence time. However, some doctors are very specific about the limitations imposed. For example, they may advise: no stairs for two weeks, no driving for one week, no sex for six weeks, etc. I believe that the best advice I can offer is to allow the level of fatigue to guide the patient. After all, patients vary in their energy level or their ability to recuperate. Until fatigue is felt, the more active the patient the better, walking being considered the best exercise. As soon as there is fatigue, the patient must stop whatever he is doing and rest. Lifting heavy objects and straining, even for a bowel movement, should be avoided for six weeks. High fluid intake, the equivalent of eight glasses of water a day, soothes urine flow. Alcohol, coffee, and spices are best avoided until recovery is complete, a period that may last two to three months.

It is not impossible to father a child after prostate surgery should one wish to try to do so. In a minority of patients, the ejaculate may shoot forward. In the majority, the ejaculate that has discharged into the bladder can be forcefully urinated out. More often, intercourse takes place on an empty bladder and, after orgasm, the ejaculate is collected from the bladder and used for insemination. The chances of a successful pregnancy are, however, remote.

When There Are Other Health Problems
Prostate enlargement occurs after middle age, a time when there are sometimes other health considerations.

What if surgery for benign enlargement has to be considered in someone who has had a heart attack? Surgery should not take place within three months of a heart attack. The risks of a repeat attack are too high. The risks do drop off somewhat after three months, but it is wisest to wait a full six months before surgery, since, at that time, the risks become indistinguishable. It is an added insurance to arrange postoperative care in an intensive care unit where heart function is closely monitored. With these precautions, patients who have had a heart attack can undergo prostate surgery just like anybody else. Patients who have had coronary bypass surgery are not at increased risk and patients who have heart valve problems have a twenty percent chance of heart complications.

Diabetic patients need careful management of their insulin, but diabetes is never a contraindication for surgery. There is, however, an increased risk of infection because the diabetic's weak bladder muscles do not allow it to empty completely.

The risk of a stroke, particularly in a patient with high blood pressure, is a concern, but even in the highest risk group with evidence of narrowed neck arteries there have not been increased attacks of strokes with prostate surgery.

Other Operations for Benign Prostate Enlargement

The enlarged prostate can also be removed through an incision made in the lower abdomen. A decision may be made to approach the prostate in this manner because the patient cannot be positioned for the procedure through the penis when, for example, there is a severe hip problem. More often, the decision is based on the size of the gland. When the prostate is very large, it may be unreasonable to expect the carving procedure through the penis to be completed within the hour.

These so-called "open" operations on the prostate take three forms. The oldest method is through a cut made into the bladder. This is an easy operation to perform, but is associated with distressing and painful bladder spasms. A second approach is through the opened capsule of the prostate. This is like incising the peel of a tangerine, placing a finger under the peel and pulling out the fruit. It is often almost as easy, and is the procedure I favor. A third approach is a cut behind the scrotum in front of the anus. I never use this method. There is a risk of damaging the nerves and I am unwilling to risk it.

These "open" operations on the prostate may also be selected because there is a need to carry out other corrective procedures at the same time. For example, it is possible to repair a blowout of the bladder, remove a large bladder stone, or even repair an inguinal hernia.

The hospitalization may be a few days longer and, as there is a cut, there is a chance of wound infection. These are minor points and, in fact, there is little difference in the postoperative course associated with these procedures compared to the more common operation through the penis.

As far as we now know, surgery is the only treatment for prostate enlargement. As frightening as surgery may be for some, prostate operations done for benign enlargement are most often quick, technically advanced, and successful. Should you need such an operation, it is wise to be mentally prepared. Awareness of what is happening to you and a positive attitude will, as in all cases of illness, aid your recovery.

QUESTIONS AND ANSWERS

Will I lose potency after the benign prostate operation?

There are very few guarantees in the biological sciences. The surgery will not affect your hormone levels, the circulation to your penis, or your nerve connections. If you had no potency problem before surgery, you are unlikely to develop impotence. If you are relatively impotent, there is about a thirty percent chance that the impotence will be worse.

How come I need a prostate operation when I've been told I have a small prostate?

It is possible that you may need an operation to improve urine flow, while another man with a large prostate may not. Patients have variable responses to discomfort. One man's agony is another man's discomfort. I suspect that when the normal outer prostate tissue is compressed by the enlarging inner tissue, some men have more elasticity in their tissue than others and they may, therefore, feel less difficulty with urination.

Are you going to use antibiotics during surgery?

Experts disagree on whether or not to use antibiotics to prevent an infection. Some feel that in the absence of a documented infection, antibiotics should not be used. Others argue that a urinary tract irritated with instruments and catheters is vulnerable to infection, and that antibiotics used before and after surgery will reduce the risk of fever, chill, and dangerous kidney infections. I use antibiotics for a short period before and after surgery.

Will I have a blood transfusion during or after the operation?

The amount of blood lost depends on a number of factors: the length of surgery, the skill of the surgeon, and the nature of the prostate

46

tissue. I will have blood available and administer it when there are dangerous changes in the cardiovascular status. You should know that as much blood is lost in the days following surgery as is lost during surgery. Do not be alarmed during this period since it only takes a little blood to color the urine alarmingly red.

What are the chances that you might find an unsuspected cancer after my prostate operation?

When there has been no suggestion of cancer on the rectal examination, there is still a ten to fifteen percent chance of an unsuspected cancer. But prostate cancer often starts in the outer part of the prostate, the part not removed in the standard carving-out process. So even when all the tissue removed shows no sign of cancer, prostate cancer can develop in subsequent years.

Will the prostate operation fix all my symptoms?

In general, if the indications were correct and the operation properly done, the symptoms will improve. If the indications for the operation were incorrect, the symptoms will not be alleviated. A scar which narrows the caliber of the urethra can occur as a consequence of an injury due to the instrument or due to the catheter. This complication will reproduce all the symptoms of an enlarged prostate. An incomplete removal of the obstructing tissue, especially of the critical tissue close to the sphincter, will leave the patient with persistent symptoms.

Will I need a repeat operation?

Repeat operations may become necessary for a number of reasons. For example, the first operation may have been terminated prematurely. This is an uncommon event, but even a quality surgeon will swallow his pride and stop, whether or not he is finished, when the safe time limit of sixty to ninety minutes has elapsed.

Another reason for a repeat operation might be the regrowth of obstructing prostate tissue. Men who have had their prostate operation at a young age, or who have the good fortune to live to a ripe old age, will have a greater chance of requiring a second operation. About fifteen percent of patients need a second operation within fifteen years.

Unlike surgery requiring a scalpel, the repeat operation is not complicated by the first because there is no obstructing scar tissue in the approach.

CANCER   If all men over fifty routinely had rectal examinations, and sample tissue from all suspicious prostates were taken out by a needle and examined under a microscope (a biopsy), there would be a dramatic change in the death rate from prostate cancer. Normally, it does not require much expertise to distinguish a malignant prostate from a benign one. While cancer feels hard like a knuckle, the normal prostate or the benign enlargement feels soft like the fleshy part of a palm. This precautionary measure will detect eighty-five to ninety percent of all early cancers. The other ten to fifteen percent do not produce the firmness that can be detected by digital rectal examination. In these instances, early diagnosis can only be made serendipitously —if there is an associated benign enlargement sufficient to encourage prostate removal as discussed in the last section. The wormlike prostate chips removed through the resectoscope and the solid mass of tissue removed with "open" surgery are routinely examined by the pathologist. The cancers undetected by digital rectal examination are usually found in this way.

When the pathologist sees cancerous changes in only one chip, or in a maximum of three chips, the disease is labeled stage A1. When cancer is detected in all the chips or in more than three chips, the disease is labeled stage A2.

Management of Stage A1 Disease
There is considerable controversy regarding how patients with stage A1 cancer of the prostate should be managed. Some doctors give the patients periodic rectal examinations and further biopsies, blood tests, and bone scans only when they suspect that the cancer is spreading. Some doctors do not distinguish A1 from A2 disease, and take out the entire prostate for A1 cancer. Many doctors go back and carve out more prostate tissue before labeling the disease A1 or A2.

Management of Stage A2 Disease
Patients with stage A2 cancer of the prostate require further treatment. Without it, the disease will spread and kill. The best treatment

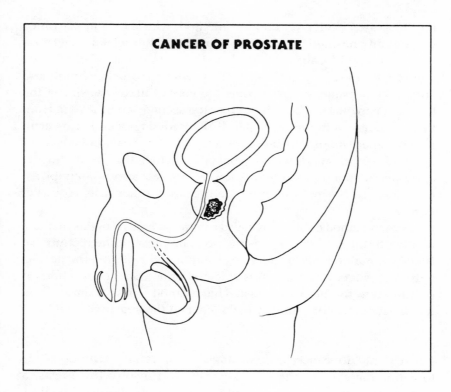

CANCER OF PROSTATE

is total surgical removal of the prostate, an operation called radical prostatectomy. Radiotherapy is considered second best, but may be the better choice for patients who are at high risk for complications with a major operation.

When cancer of the prostate is suspected upon rectal examination, but the examining finger does not detect disease in adjacent organs, the disease is designated a stage B lesion. The B lesion covers a category that varies from a tiny nodule smaller than a pea to that involving the entire prostate, sometimes further categorized as stage B2. The diagnosis is confirmed by biopsy.

Prostate Biopsy
Prostate biopsy can be done in different ways. One way is to make a surgical exposure with a cut behind the scrotum in front of the rectum. Another way is to stick a needle through the skin at a point between the scrotum and the anus with a finger in the rectum guid-

ing the way. I prefer yet another method, which I do in my office without an anesthetic. I place my gloved and lubricated finger into the rectum and localize the hard spot in the prostate. Then I slide a biopsy needle along my finger. The needle pierces the rectum and enters the prostate, where it collects a core of tissue the size of the lead in a pencil. The procedure takes ten seconds and the pain from the prostate is a momentary jab. If the pathologist finds cancer in the specimen, no further biopsy is necessary. If the pathologist cannot find cancer, there will be concern whether the needle hit the appropriate spot or not. It may even require repeating—an unpleasant prospect, but not any more painful than other tests requiring needles.

Another method of biopsy is called aspiration biopsy. In this method, a much thinner needle pierces the prostate through the rectum. No tissue is obtained, but by applying suction and agitating the needle, a droplet is recovered which is smeared on a microscopic slide for examination by the pathologist. This method is less accurate, and a confirmatory "core" biopsy is done when the smear is positive.

Staging
The patient with cancer is then "staged." This is, an attempt is made to define the extent of the disease. This will involve three tests: a bone scan, a blood test, and an ultrasound examination of the liver and spleen.

The bone scan is a radioisotope study. A chemical that emits gamma rays is injected into the vein and will localize in bone cells. A picture of the radiation emitted from the chemical is thus like a picture of a skeleton. When cancer is present in the bone, it shows up as extra dots on the picture or as extra blanks. Arthritic joints and bones previously fractured show extra dots as well, sometimes confusing the interpretation. A normal X ray of the same area is often correlated with the bone scan results to clarify the problem. The radiation from the test and X rays is minimal and the interpretation often boils down to a judgment call aided by the results of the blood test done with it to stage the disease.

The blood is tested for an enzyme called prostatic acid phosphatase, specifically secreted by the cancerous prostate cells. Unfortunately, this enzyme cannot be detected in the blood until the disease has moved well beyond the prostate. In the majority of cases, elevated levels mean that the disease has spread, even when the rectal examination suggests confinement. This enzyme can become elevated as well when part of the prostate suddenly loses its blood supply, a condition called infarct of the prostate.

The ultrasound test of the liver and spleen tells us if the cancer has spread into these organs.

After involving the lymph nodes, eighty percent of prostate cancers spread first to bones, and twenty percent spread first to the liver. Thus in staging the disease, the doctor is guided by a battery of tests, not by one test alone. Accurate staging is the backbone of proper management. It is very important because drastically different decisions are based on the results of staging. And, incidentally, the amount of radiation used for these tests is inconsequential: like worrying about the wallpaper when the house is on fire.

Management of Stage B and A2 Disease—Operable Cancer

When the cancer is confined to the prostate, the objective is total eradication of the disease. Traditionally, three methods competed as the method of choice: radical surgery, radiotherapy, and radioisotope therapy.

Radical Surgery Total surgical removal of the prostate is a major undertaking. The operation may take four to five hours and there are risks of serious complications. Besides the normal risk factors of every major operation—chances of pneumonia, wound infection, blood clots in the legs that may migrate to the lungs—there are risk factors peculiar to this procedure. There is a ten percent chance of losing urine control, a three percent chance of dying from complications, and what used to be a ninety-nine percent chance of impotence. These figures are changing dramatically in recent years. For example, I have not yet had a patient who is totally incontinent after surgery, and with the recently introduced nerve-sparing operation developed by Dr. Patrick Walsh of Johns Hopkins University, the chances of recovering potency are fifty to ninety percent.

The operation starts with removal of the pelvic lymph nodes because when prostate cancer spreads, it always spreads first to the pelvic lymph nodes. To date, we have no foolproof way of telling if the lymph nodes are involved without first actually doing the surgery. The naked eye cannot tell if the lymph node harbors cancer or not. (The CT scan can detect lymph nodes that are larger than

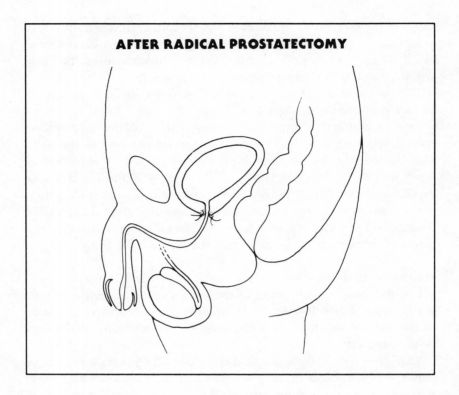

AFTER RADICAL PROSTATECTOMY

two centimeters, but smaller nodes can be cancerous.) Surgery is done and the excised lymph nodes are sent to the pathologist, who quickly freezes the specimen, slices it, stains it, and examines it under the microscope. I rely on the frozen section reading. If there is cancer in the lymph nodes, I abandon the operation because the chances are that the cancer is in other parts of the body and thus the disease cannot be totally eliminated by surgery. I proceed with the prostate removal when the pathologist gives me a report that there is no cancer in the lymph nodes.

Prostate removal is one of the more difficult operations because the area is bloody, surgery takes place in the depth of the wound, and the delicate, pencil-thin urethra has to be rejoined to the wide open neck of the bladder. All this has to occur without damage to the cobweb-like nerves that lie just behind the prostate if potency is to be preserved.

The operation starts with the patient placed flat on his back and

52

anesthetized. The skin from the nipples to midthigh is scrubbed with surgical soap and painted with an antiseptic solution. Sterile drapes cover the body except for the lower abdomen. A catheter is placed into the bladder.

I make a vertical incision that extends from the belly button to the pubic bone. I split the muscle below the skin in the midline. I stretch the muscle open and am then into the site for the proposed surgery.

I dissect out the pelvic lymph nodes and send them to the pathologist for frozen section examination. Then I free the prostate gland on both sides and clamp and tie the large vein in front of the prostate. I can now see where the urethra enters the prostate. I cut the top of the urethra, exposing the catheter inside, and make a stitch on either side of the urethra so it won't pull apart. I take the catheter out and cut completely through the urethra. The prostate is still fixed to its bed behind, and to the bladder on top. I gently dissect the back wall of the prostate upward toward the bladder, protecting the nerve that is necessary for potency. I then cut the prostate away from the bladder. Next I cut away the vas and the blood supply from the back of the prostate wall. The seminal vesicles are dissected so that they can be removed with the prostate. Only now can I remove the prostate. After the prostate removal, I fit the larger bladder to the urethral opening by stitching it smaller and fix it to the urethra with four stitches, using the two stitches previously placed. A Foley catheter is put into the bladder, tubes are placed in the wound for spilled urine and blood, and the wound is closed.

Radical prostatectomy is very major surgery and, in my estimation, one of the most challenging technical procedures because the operation involves delicate reconstruction of the urinary tract. When there is meticulous attention to detail, there are fewer complications, and continence and potency are preserved. In recent years (1985 and thereafter), surgery has become the treatment of choice for stage B and A2 prostate cancer because the results are superior to radiotherapy or radioisotope therapy.

Radiotherapy With radiotherapy, powerful gamma rays are directed at the prostate gland from many directions. These rays kill cancer cells more than they do normal cells, but the distinction is fuzzy. Thus when radiation hits the skin in substantial amounts, the skin turns brown and hard. When radiation irritates the lower bowel, there can be cramps, diarrhea, and pain. Radiation injury to the bladder can contract the bladder, causing frequent need for urination. It can also cause easy bleeding from the bladder lining.

Despite these potential problems to the skin, bowel, or bladder, most patients seldom suffer, and many are helped.

However, while the cancer is contained, it is often not eradicated. Biopsies taken after curative courses of radiotherapy show cancer in the original site. Nevertheless, the cancer *is* largely contained and radiotherapy to the prostate is less hazardous and toxic to the body than radiotherapy to the lungs or abdomen.

Radioisotope Therapy The radioisotope treatment was pioneered at the Sloan-Kettering Cancer Center in New York City. In this operation, the prostate gland is dissected free from its surrounding tissue and, instead of being removed, radioactive pellets are inserted into it. This takes advantage of the powerful gamma rays without risking their complications. But this does require fairly major surgery, and the cancer is contained rather than cured.

I treat my patients having stage B and A2 disease with radical prostatectomy. In cases in which there is a medical contraindication to surgery, I offer them radiotherapy. I am not convinced that radioisotope implantation is sufficiently superior to external beam therapy to justify the rigors of the surgery involved.

Stage C Disease

When the examining rectal finger detects cancer spread to the seminal vesicle, bladder, or urethra, the disease is labeled stage C. Stage C disease is often found by a CT scan, an X ray that shows a mass of two centimeters or more.

Management of Stage C Disease

Stage C cancer of the prostate is managed like a stage B or a stage D. That is, on the presumption that the cancer is only in the prostate, it is managed like a B and radical surgery is done. Occasionally, we see with hindsight that the disease has spread beyond the prostate and is, in fact, a C. When we know beforehand that the disease has spread beyond the prostate, but not to distant sites, most urologists manage the patient with hormonal manipulation, as if he had stage D disease, or with a course of radiotherapy.

Stage D Disease

When cancer has spread into the lymph nodes or beyond, it is labeled stage D. This category is further subdivided into D1 or D2, depending on whether the cancer has spread only into the lymph nodes of the pelvis or beyond. In stage D2 disease, the cancer has spread beyond the pelvic lymph nodes, the bone scan is positive, and the enzyme released by the prostatic cancer cell is elevated. Unfortunately, the majority of patients with cancer of the prostate are diagnosed at this stage.

Management of Stage D Disease

The majority (eighty percent) of prostate cancers are hormone dependent. This means that the cancer is stimulated by a certain hormonal environment and is inhibited by another hormonal environment. Dr. Charles Huggins of the University of Chicago was the first to show this in 1941.

Prostate cancer is stimulated by the male hormone, testosterone. Thus removal of the testicles, the main source of testosterone production, can cause dramatic resolution of the cancer. An almost identical effect can be achieved by the administration of the female hormone, diethylstilbestrol (DES), by mouth; or by daily injections of a drug that acts on the master gland (pituitary), inhibiting production of testosterone. Removal of the testicles is a minor surgical undertaking, but can be psychologically devastating. In my experience, the psychology is overrated. Patients with cancer are anxious to get help, not preserve body image or potency. Virtually all my patients faced with D type cancer learn to accept surgical removal of the testicles. The occasional patient opts for insertion of the testicular prosthesis: these are soft plastic balls that resemble the testicles in size and consistency.

The hormone testosterone is also produced by the adrenal gland. To counteract this, another pill, an antiandrogen called Flutamide, has been added to the treatment regime. I believe this will improve survival. Hormonal manipulation will not improve the lot of prostate cancers that are not hormone dependent, but it is the treatment of choice for eighty percent of advanced prostate cancers.

The combination of testicle removal or estrogen or pituitary gland antagonist plus Flutamide may be achieved by one medication called

Cyproperone Acetate (Androcur). The dual effect of this pill is sound, but long-term results are not yet fully established.

All patients are followed with periodic bone scans and determinations of enzyme levels released from prostatic cancer cells. Most patients (eighty percent) will show improvement in the way they feel, in the bone pain, and in weight loss. There will be a corresponding improvement in the bone scan picture and the enzyme level. Sometimes the remissions are lifelong, sometimes less.

Prostate cancer is common, but curable if diagnosed early, and controllable even with a late diagnosis. More patients with this disease die from natural causes than from an uncontrolled progression of the disease.

QUESTIONS AND ANSWERS

How good is the ultrasound test for diagnosing cancer of the prostate?

An ultrasound examination of the prostate can suggest cancer before the disease is apparent in a rectal examination, and I have little doubt that ultrasound will become the test of choice for early diagnosis. The test is in its infancy. Enthusiasts are guilty of exaggerated claims, while critics are negative because they lack expertise. Pioneering centers, such as the one at the University of Michigan at Ann Arbor, Michigan, can confidently detect cancers that are a few millimeters in size and can guide the biopsy needle to the spot. Many other medical centers in the United States and Europe feel that their rate of false positives (images that show cancer on the ultrasound test but are not confirmed by biopsy) and false negatives (cancers that are absent on the ultrasound test but present in the surgically removed specimen) is much too high to establish ultrasound as a valid screening test. Undoubtedly, refinement of the machinery and further experience will clarify the issue.

How is an ultrasound examination of the prostate done?
The patient is asked to lie on his side. A probe, about the size of a finger, is inserted into the rectum. The tip of the probe is covered with a condom-like sac filled with water. When the probe is activated, it is like turning on a flashlight of sound waves. The prostate is seen as the sound waves bounce off it. The early cancer shows

up like a black hole on a white background. A needle that is fixed to the probe can, then, be guided through the skin and into the spot, while the gland is under observation. The entire procedure may take ten to fifteen minutes.

Aren't there any blood tests that diagnose prostate cancer?

There is an enzyme, called prostatic acid phosphatase, produced by the prostate cancer cells. But this enzyme can only be detected in the blood when the cancer has spread beyond the prostate. Blood tests are good for disease control but not for early detection.

Isn't it true that radioactive seeds can be placed in the prostate without opening the skin?

This technique is being explored in Sweden and holds much promise. A needle similar to a biopsy needle, mounted on an ultrasound probe, places radioactive pellets into the prostate. I suspect that when early disease is diagnosed by the ultrasound test this will become the treatment of choice.

Even if the cancer has spread beyond the prostate, shouldn't you remove the prostate anyway?

The Mayo Clinic is exploring radical prostatectomy, plus removal of the testicles, in cancers that have spread into the lymph nodes but not beyond. The long-term results of this approach are not yet known. If it is true, as is generally accepted, that new deposits of cancer can come only from the original site, there may be some merit to this approach. I have used the Mayo approach in treating some of my patients, but time alone will tell whether or not it is justified. Critics of this approach will argue that equal or better survival results may be achieved with hormonal treatment only.

Do I need hormone pills after a radical prostatectomy?

If the surgery was for a cure and a cure has been effected, no further treatment is necessary. Every six months, follow-up tests are done. These include blood enzyme levels, bone scan, and a chest X ray. If there is evidence that the tumor is recurring (elevated prostatic acid phosphatase or a positive bone scan), hormonal treatment will be necessary to contain the cancer. This is done either by removing the testicles or administering hormone pills.

Can the pathologist be wrong in his diagnosis of cancer?
This is most unlikely. When the pathologist is uncertain, he describes his misgivings and examines more sections of the specimen. When the pathologist says it's a cancer, it is, unfortunately, a cancer.

INFECTION Of the three common maladies afflicting the prostate gland—namely, benign enlargement, cancer, and prostatitis—the last is the most frequently misdiagnosed, mistreated, and misunderstood.

First of all, there is no clear understanding of why bacterial prostatitis occurs. We know that an invasion of the bowel bacteria through the bloodstream and into the prostate causes infection and inflammation of the prostate gland. This describes the route of infection, but we don't know why prostatitis occurs in some people and not in others. There seems to be no sexual association. People who have not had sex get bacterial prostatitis as often as those who have.

Although a venereal cause is remotely possible, the microorganisms associated with prostatitis are usually not of that variety. The vast majority of cases of prostatitis have no sexual implications. Like bacterial infections in other organs—tonsillitis, bronchitis, or meningitis, for example—microorganisms settle in a particular part of the body because there is a specific predisposition and, sometimes, for no good reason at all. The prostate may be predisposed to infection in someone who bounces up and down on his bottom against a hard surface. Indeed, prostatitis has long been called the "jeep driver's disease." Constipation has also been suggested as a predisposing factor. By and large, however, no specific causative factor can be found. In my practice, I have found patients uniformly agreeing on one thing: "Yes, I have been working too hard and not getting much sleep. And yes, I have been under considerable stress of late." In other words, prostatitis is a disease of our times.

Whatever the reason, bowel bacteria, most often *Escherichia coli*, settle into the prostate. The illness then takes one of two forms. Either there is an acute illness with high fever, chills, prostration, and difficulty with urine flow: acute prostatitis; or there is a vague malaise, itchy urethra, discomfort in the area behind the scrotum and in front of the anus, called the perineum, and perhaps some discomfort on urination: chronic prostatitis.

Acute Prostatitis

Acute prostatitis may require hospitalization, intravenous fluids, and powerful antibiotics, but the clinical course of the illness is relatively short, with complete and total recovery. The diagnosis is not difficult to establish: microorganisms are almost always seen in the urine and blood. A routine culture of the urine and blood confirms the diagnosis. Traditionally, medical students are taught not to subject patients to repeated rectal examinations. Upon the first examination, the infected prostate will be hot and tender, and pressing on it is like squeezing an infected pimple: there is a risk of pushing microorganisms into the bloodstream.

Once in a while a patient will not respond to even the most powerful drugs, and there will be persistent high fever. An abscess of the prostate is likely. This condition is best treated by allowing the abscess to drain into the urinary passage. The instrument that was used to carve out the prostate (a resectoscope) is used to create the drainage.

Despite the ominous nature of some of the phrases used here (powerful drugs, high fever, surgical drainage, etc.) acute prostatitis is almost always certainly curable.

Chronic Prostatitis

Chronic prostatitis, on the other hand, can linger so long it has driven men to utter despair, suicide sometimes not far from their minds. Constant low back pain, a continual urgent need to urinate, disabling discomfort in the rectum or lower abdomen, loss of libido, and impotence are persistent symptoms that may combine to make life seem not worth living.

But chronic prostatitis is frequently misdiagnosed. A patient may be saddled with the diagnosis with little supporting evidence. He may have some discomfort that he localizes to the area near the prostate; he may find urination uncomfortable and frequent. However, these symptoms may all arise from anxiety and have no basis in a physical disorder.

Bona fide chronic prostatitis can also be misdiagnosed. The doctor may presume he is dealing with a psychosomatic disorder and may not take the steps necessary to establish the diagnosis.

The diagnosis cannot be made from the history, nor from examination of the urine. Only by carrying out a vigorous prostatic massage with the gloved and lubricated finger in the rectum, expressing fluid from the urethra, and examining it under the microscope, can the doctor, in my estimation, rule in or rule out the diagnosis of chronic prostatitis. If a patient has the disorder, the doctor will see more than fifteen white blood cells under a microscope that is set at forty times magnification. Patients without the disorder will have less than fifteen white blood cells. Period. Other tests are sometimes proposed—culture of the urine after massage, culture of the ejaculate, a test to see how the fluid in the blood separates from the cells—but these tests are much less important. I am guided strictly by what I see under the microscope, especially when I see the white blood cells in clumps.

The massage is distressful and often painful for the patient. I am not at all convinced that the prostate constitutes an erogenous zone. On the other hand, there is not much doubt that the anus might be.

Treatment consists of general measures and specific measures. General measures include: high fluid intake to flush the system, hot tub baths to encourage more circulation to the area, and an active sex life to accomplish what periodic prostatic massage will do. Alcohol, coffee, and spices should be restricted if not eliminated. They are all irritants, causing tissue swelling, and their use is like adding gasoline to fire.

What the doctor does specifically is to prescribe antibiotics. The problem is that there is a blood-prostate barrier: few antibacterials diffuse from the bloodstream into the prostate. Two products that do are the trimethoprim-sulfamethoxozole combination called Septra or Bactrim, and erythromycin. Erythromycin is not very effective against bowel microorganisms like *E. coli*, which is the most common bacterial cause of prostatitis. Its efficacy can be improved by adding baking soda to the regime. The baking soda helps to make the body fluids more alkaline, a better environment for the drug. The trimethoprim-sulfamethoxazole combination is the most effective and most commonly used medication. The usual dosage is a double-strength pill taken twice a day.

Second-generation tetracyclines, like minocycline (Minocin) or doxycycline (Vibramycin), are considered effective by some experts. The ordinary tetracycline has to be taken on an empty stomach to be fully effective, loses potency when taken with milk, can cause teeth discoloration, and can create a problem if the patient is exposed to direct sunlight, something equivalent to snow blindness. All these problems are eliminated by the new generation of the drug. But it seldom eradicates chronic prostatitis and is therefore not the drug of choice.

The quinolone family of drugs, such as norfloxacin (Noroxin), may prove helpful, but it has not yet been sufficiently time-tested.

Chronic prostatitis has been likened to a fire in a haystack. The fire can appear to be out but it is still smoldering underneath. The drug treatment has to be long and protracted: six to twelve weeks that can stretch into a year and longer. I continue with the drugs and the restrictions until the prostatic fluid is clear. It does happen but not often. Frequently, the prostatic fluid will clear, but the patient will have a lingering malaise. At this point, supportive psychotherapy becomes important.

I do not even object if the patient wants to try a little black magic—multivitamins or zinc, for example. The rationale for the use of zinc is based on the finding that there is more zinc in the prostate gland than in any other organ in the body. The thinking has been that if there is a problem in the prostate, there may be a need for this metal. What harm can there be in trying it? In fact, there is scientific evidence that in the presence of zinc deficiency, supplemental zinc administration will speed up healing. The zinc has to be administered by injection, though. There is no evidence that zinc in pill form has ever affected healing.

There is little role for surgery in the treatment of chronic prostatitis. Sometimes, a patient will convince his doctor to resort to the knife, so desperate is his plight. But there is no assurance that a radical prostatectomy will cure the patient of his symptoms.

A CAUTIONARY NOTE It is remarkable, that a gland that is normally so small, a gland the size of a walnut, can be the source of so much male distress.

The capacity for orgasm is not lost after surgery for benign enlargement but can be lost when the prostate gland is removed totally or is badly diseased. Benign enlargement can choke the flow of urine; cancer often defies early diagnosis and, when advanced, can kill; and infection is often impervious to antimicrobial treatment.

A prudent man will cut down on those items that appear to irritate the gland, namely alcohol, coffee, and spices. He will drink more water, eat more fresh vegetables and fruit, consume more fish and white poultry meat at the expense of red meat. He will submit to regular rectal examination and, perhaps, to transrectal prostatic ultrasound exams when they become established. And he will maintain an active sex life.

How can my problem be in the prostate when I feel all the discomfort at the head of the penis?

Branches of the pudendal nerve go to the prostate and also to the head of the penis. When the prostate is irritated, it stimulates this nerve and the sensation is felt, simultaneously, at the head of the penis. This is similar to the process whereby pain in the heart is felt in the shoulder tip, since the heart and shoulder tip are supplied also by the same nerve. This process is called "referred pain."

If I keep having prostatitis, why can't my prostate just be cut out?

Carving out the inner part of the prostate, as is done for benign enlargement, will leave behind an infected bed. Prostatitis will not be cured, the healing process will be prolonged, and there is a high risk that a scar will close down the juncture between the bladder and the prostate. The only surgery that might help is total removal of the prostate, as is done when there is early cancer. In the past, such surgery was seldom considered because there was a one hundred percent certainty of impotence and a ten percent risk of losing control over the bladder. The recent development of a method of radical prostatectomy, which preserves potency and has a very low risk of incontinence, may encourage reconsideration of surgical treatment for disabling chronic prostatitis.

Can prostatitis affect potency?

At the height of the problem, all men are impotent or are anxious about their sexuality. They feel miserable and are often afraid that either they will not be potent or they will transmit the problem to their partner. When the symptoms have subsided, most men recover full potency. Some men report reduced potency, but it is difficult to know whether the problem is physical or psychological.

Can I give my partner a sexually transmitted disease if I have prostatitis?

It is theoretically possible to transmit the bowel bacteria of prostatitis from one person to another through the semen. In practice, this is seldom a problem since there are not enough bacteria to cause an infection in the vagina. Nevertheless, I suggest a condom for the first two weeks after the treatment has started. After two weeks, I think the condom is probably unnecessary. I have never yet had a man's partner come to me with an infection, but I must confess that I am not certain what is happening in the private lives of the people concerned.

If coffee is bad for me when I have prostatitis, can I use the decaffeinated brand?

Coffee contains over one hundred chemical ingredients and caffeine, per se, does not appear to be the only irritant. Tea, which contains caffeine, is much less of an irritant.

Why don't I take twice as many pills as you prescribed?

It won't help. The chances of stomach and bowel upset would increase and the prognosis would not improve. If you are going to second-guess the doctor, it would make more sense to prolong the duration of treatment.

5 INFERTILITY

It is generally agreed that ten to fifteen percent of all unions are barren. In other words, one out of every eight marriages is childless. Infertility is, unfortunately, much more common than most people realize.

Which partner is responsible for the infertility? In my experience, it is one-third male related, one-third female related, and one-third unknown. To find out which partner is infertile, exhaustive tests used to be carried out on the woman before the man was considered for study. This bias has been changing in recent years because investigation of the male is easier and less traumatic. There is no doubt that an infertility investigation should start with the man.

INVESTIGATION OF THE MALE Infertility is a condition rather than a malady. Indeed, in most instances, there are no other health problems: there is no urinary symptom, no sexual malfunction, no suggestion of anything else being wrong.

The medical history seldom yields any hints as to why there might be an infertility problem. What might be pertinent is a history of mumps, which can destroy the testicle after puberty, but mumps usually affect only one testicle. An inguinal hernia repair can also choke the blood flow to the testicle, particularly if the repair is tight. I have seen a number of testicles damaged by hernia repair, but infertility is seldom a consequence since surgery is normally done on only one side. Certain chemicals, like lead, are known to be toxic to the testicles, but I have never seen a case of infertility attributable to chemical exposure. On the other hand, I have seen cases of testicular damage due to radiotherapy, or due to certain antibacterial drugs such as nitrofurantoin, which is prescribed for urinary tract infection. Damage due to drugs, however, is usually reversible after the drug is stopped.

The Physical Exam

There is one physical finding that a doctor looks for specifically: a varicose vein in the scrotum, usually on the left, called a varicocele. Ten percent of the male population have a left-sided varicocele, and in the absence of pain or discomfort, little fuss is made of it. But with the presence of an infertility problem, the finding of a varicocele can be meaningful because correction can improve the fertility status (as will be discussed below).

On rare occasions there can be a startling physical finding. For example, the vas deferens might be missing. This is the tube that conducts the sperm from the testicles to a storage depot. While a man can be born without the vas, he will be normal in every other way, his testicles and hormone levels being quite normal, and he will have no disability other than infertility. In effect, he has the equivalent of a vasectomy. It is not known why such a condition should occur. (It is one of the possible consequences of diethylstilbestrol [DES] taken by the mother during pregnancy, but usually such a history is not known.) So far, we have no method to reverse this condition. In other rare cases, the patient's testicles may appear extraordinarily small and perhaps a little firmer than usual. Furthermore, he may be lanky with rather long arms. Such a combination suggests Klinefelter's syndrome—an aberration of the chromosomes associated with infertility. Another uncommon finding might be an absent testicle on one side and an apparent disorder in the remaining one. There is also the possibility that a man might have breast tissue more like that of a female, raising concern about testis cancer, or might have lumpy bumps along the vas, which is seen in tuberculosis. But the majority of men with an apparent infertility problem have completely normal sexual organs.

What *is* unusual is their telltale history: an active sex life, no contraceptive protection, and no pregnancy.

Semen Analysis

The critical test necessary to define the problem is the examination of the ejaculate: semen analysis. Different laboratories may offer different directions on how the specimen should be harvested, but certain instructions are standard. There must be a three- to four-day period of abstinence from sex, the ejaculate must be collected in a clean bottle, and it must be examined within two hours. Specimens collected in a condom or stored in a refrigerator cannot be interpreted.

The hospital laboratory where I work schedules men to come at prearranged dates, provides them with a container, and asks them to produce a specimen by masturbation. I was unaware of any problems until one patient complained to me of his ordeal: "I was thoroughly embarrassed. . . . You certainly did not prepare me. . . . Imagine, a young lady passes me a jar and tells me where the bathroom is located. The tiny closet toilet is ill-kept and, in fact, not very private. I don't know whether those things affect the results or not, but I can tell you it was not a pleasant experience." I commiserated with him and acknowledged his complaint, but insisted that when it comes to the hospital, modesty is left at the front door.

I have had to deal with patients who insisted that their religion did not allow them to masturbate, those who wanted to bring their wives and be provided with a place to copulate, and those who insisted on collecting the specimen at home and arrived with a jar containing a fluid-soaked condom. In general, however, semen analysis raises no more problems than any other laboratory test.

As a rule, I request three separate analyses of the collected semen.

The detailed reports from the lab include volume, pH (degree of acidity or alkalinity), color, presence or absence of fructose, bacteria, white blood cells, etc. All these aspects may be relevant, but what is most important is the number of active sperm per unit volume.

A specimen from a fertile man will show a high sperm count, over fifty and up to two hundred million per milliliter. More than sixty percent of the sperm will have normal forms (not double-headed, tiny-headed, or giant-headed). And most of them will be vigorously swimming in a straight line. Specimens from an infertile man are likely to show less than twenty million sperm per milliliter, with many dead and abnormal forms, and a larger percentage swimming languidly in circles.

When the semen analysis reports an absence of fructose, it means that the man was born without seminal vesicles. There is no corrective measure for this abnormality.

When the semen analysis detects sperm, but of a lesser count or vitality, blood tests for hormones are undertaken. The hormones tested are LH (luteinizing hormone), FSH (follicle-stimulating hormone), testosterone, and, sometimes, prolactin.

Hormone Tests

If there is a problem with LH or testosterone, appropriate replacement therapy may help solve the problem. If the prolactin is abnormal, it is suggested that there may be a problem in the pituitary gland. But the most frequent finding is a very high reading of FSH, signaling irreversible damage to the testicles. I take the reading of the FSH seriously. The FSH is a hormone secreted by the pituitary gland in response to the number and vitality of the sperm production by the testicles. If sperm production is proceeding normally, the FSH output is at a normal level. When there is no sperm, or few sperm, the FSH level rises in response. If the FSH is high, I stop further investigation and counsel the patient that science has no solution for his condition at this time. If the FSH is normal and the ejaculate shows no sperm, I stick a tiny tuberculin needle into the structure located behind the testicle and suck out a drop of fluid. This tissue, which drains the sperm from the testicle, is called the epididymis. The drop is examined under the microscope and checked for the presence of sperm. If sperm are present, an exploration for a blockage is recommended. When the FSH is normal, I keep encouraging the patient to keep his hopes up, even if he is beginning to despair.

The test for hormone levels has made biopsy of the testis obsolete, as far as I am concerned. Testis biopsy is still being done, but I see no merit in it.

In the case of a man, the investigation for infertility is really quite simple. It takes no more than a few minutes to ask the pertinent questions, another few minutes to carry out the examination, and another moment for the tests.

When no abnormality is detected in the semen analysis, and the patient is otherwise well, the investigation of the male partner stops right there. I advise the couple that I can detect nothing wrong and that investigation of the wife, if not underway, should now commence.

INVESTIGATION OF THE FEMALE A woman concerned about infertility is seen by a gynecologist. Although I am not a gynecologist, I will try to explain what is involved.

During their reproductive years, women periodically shed the lining of the uterus, which has been prepared to accept a fertilized egg. This process of shedding or bleeding is menstruation, and the cyclic occurrence is called the menstrual cycle. The entire process is controlled by the pituitary hormones LH and FSH working in harmony with estrogen and progesterone—hormones produced by the ovary.

When all systems are working normally, menstruation occurs on an average of every twenty-eight days. During such a cycle, the egg is being released from the ovary on the fourteenth day, and if intercourse takes place on or about that day, conception is possible. If menstruation is occurring every twenty-one days, the release of the egg is still likely about fourteen days before the beginning of the next menstruation. Thus in all cases, the fertile period can be determined by counting backward but can only be guessed by counting forward.

When there is an infertility problem and the man is not the cause, the gynecologist does a number of tests.

He or she may scrape the inner lining of the uterus, and give these scrapings to the pathologist to check the components of the "soil." Blood and urine samples may be taken at particular times of the menstrual cycle to check the level of the hormones. The Fallopian tubes may be checked for blockage by passing through gas or chemicals that can be X-rayed. The Fallopian tube normally accepts the egg released by the ovary and conducts it into the uterus. It is during this trip that the egg becomes fertilized by the upward-swimming sperm. The fertilized egg normally descends into the uterus, but if it becomes embedded in the wall of the tube the result is a life-threatening ectopic pregnancy. The Fallopian tube can expand only so far, and when that limit is exceeded, it ruptures. Normally, the fertilized egg will travel through the Fallopian tube and embed itself in the uterus.

The gynecologist may request daily temperature readings because

68

most women have a slight rise in their temperature when the egg is released from the ovary. Finally, the gynecologist may want to pass an instrument through the skin just under the belly button and into the abdomen, to examine the ovary and, sometimes, to extract an egg about to be released. This test is called a laparoscopy.

It is thus apparent that the investigation of the woman for infertility is more potentially injurious to the body than the investigation in the male, and that is why I recommend looking at the man first.

The Postcoital Test

Some infertility experts will insist upon a postcoital test even before a regular semen analysis. The woman is asked to report immediately after intercourse. The ejaculate is suctioned out with the cervical mucus and examined. If all the sperm are dead or immobilized, a search can be launched for the causative factors, such as sperm-killing antibodies, particularly if the regular semen analysis is normal. The timing of the postcoital test is critical: it is only valid if it is done during the woman's fertile period.

TREATMENT OF MALE INFERTILITY Often, a man is referred to me with a normally healthy partner and a normal medical history, physical, and semen analysis. This is not an uncommon scenario, and under these circumstances I recommend the following regime:

I encourage intercourse every three to four days. No more, no less. I point out that in different studies carried out, largely on prisoner volunteers, sperm count was best when ejaculation took place every fourth day and sperm vitality was best with ejaculation every three days.

At mid-cycle, when pregnancy might be possible, I advise insemination of only the first jet that comes out. After the first jet, the man should withdraw and discard the rest. The first portion of the ejaculate is the most powerful; the rest only dilutes the fluid and reduces the chances of pregnancy. I suggest that during each menstrual cycle there can be no more than two or three chances for pregnancy: when intercourse is within forty-eight hours of ovulation, and if the frequency of intercourse is maintained at intervals of three to four days.

I may ask the couple to have intercourse with condom protection for a six-month period. The rationale for this recommendation is as follows. For reasons that may never be resolved, the woman may have developed antibodies that kill or immobilize sperm. Testing for this possibility is rather expensive and often inaccurate. When antibodies are found, the traditional treatment has been a condom for six months, immunosuppression with cortisone, and instillation of the ejaculate into the uterus. These treatments are largely experimental, and successful outcomes have been few and far between. I put my patients on vitamin C, five hundred milligrams per day. Vitamin C is a reducing agent. It removes oxygen from a chemical reaction and may thus counteract the action of the antibodies. No harm can come from taking this vitamin at this dosage.

Tight jockey shorts, particularly nylon-type bikini briefs, should be discarded in favor of loose, cotton boxer shorts. The testicles are meant to hang loose, away from the body, so that they are maintained at a temperature four degrees lower than body temperature. For similar reasons, hot baths and saunas should be avoided.

After doing all that, I suggest we wait one year and meet again if pregnancy has not occurred.

Varicocele Ligation
When the semen analysis shows a low count, and when sperm are not moving vigorously, I hope to find a varicocele. If the distended vein is not immediately obvious, I try to induce it by asking the patient to force down as if straining for a bowel movement. The male anatomy is predisposed to the formation of a left-sided varicocele. The vein draining the left testicle empties into the renal vein, a foot and a half or two feet away. The column of blood appears to be too heavy for the one-way valves, and so destroys them. The end result is a distended vein with incompetent valves—a varicocele. The problem is less likely on the right side because it drains lower into the vena cava (the main venous trunk). If the varicocele is present or can be induced, surgical correction is recommended.

Surgery to correct a varicocele is a minor operation. It can be done on an outpatient basis, but I prefer to admit my patient. Under a regional or general anesthetic, a one-inch cut is made at the level of the prominence of the pelvic bone, about an inch from the margin of the bone. The muscles under the skin are split, the bowel envelope is pushed away, and the swollen vein coming from the testicle is identified. Occasionally, another vein nearby, called the inferior epigastric vein, can be mistaken for the testicular vein. This error can be prevented by tugging on the testicle—the testicular vein will move; the epigastric vein will not. This simple maneuver prevents accidental interruption of the wrong vein, an accident that I have been called upon to correct a number of times. A small segment of the testicular vein is removed. The wound is then closed, and most patients can be discharged the following day.

Why a distended vein in only the left testicle should cause an infertility problem is not clear. A long-standing varicocele does appear to shrivel the testicle. It has been argued that the extra amounts of warm blood due to the distended vein heat up the testicle and cause the damage. Others have suggested that it is some waste product from the kidney or adrenal gland that normally would not get down to the testicle that does the harm. Such a factor has not been identified. Why a disorder that affects one testicle should interfere with fertility, presumably a product of both testicles, remains unresolved.

Nevertheless, this simple operation does appear to improve sperm count and vitality. Different hospitals report successful pregnancy in twenty-five to fifty percent of patients who have varicocele ligation. The only other operation that might help infertility is unblocking a blockage, like a vasectomy reversal. This will be considered elsewhere.

Drug Treatment

Finally, if the sperm count is low but the FSH is normal, I try clomiphene citrate, a drug that stimulates greater release of FSH and LH from the pituitary gland. Half a pill, or twenty-five milligrams, is taken by mouth every day for approximately four months. If there is improvement in the sperm count, the drug is continued; if there is no substantial change, the drug is stopped.

I have not used any other drugs. Some experts feel that they can improve sperm count by administering testosterone for a period and then suddenly stopping. A rebound surge of sperm production is the hope. I am not convinced that it works nor that it is free of potential harm. Pergonal, a drug prepared from the urine of postmenopausal women and containing FSH, and bromocriptine (Parlodel) which inhibits the release of prolactin, may have a place in the treatment, but I am not convinced that they have a role in male infertility (although their role in the female treatment is better established).

TREATMENT OF FEMALE INFERTILITY Some of the advice offered women, such as that offered men, has little basis in established scientific studies. The following are what I consider reasonable recommendations:

It is reasonable to ask women to lie flat on their backs for fifteen minutes or so after intercourse. This may help prevent spillage of the ejaculate.

If the postcoital test done at the right time suggests difficulty with sperm penetration, estrogen administered on days ten through fourteen may improve the permeability of the cervical mucus. Twenty micrograms of estradiol is considered an appropriate dosage.

If the egg is not being released from the ovary, there are a number of drugs that can be employed to aid ovulation.

1. Cortisone, or prednisone at a small daily dosage, reduces the male hormone level and helps induce ovulation.

2. Clomiphene citrate stimulates FSH production and thus can initiate ovulation. A fifty-milligram tablet is administered from day five to day nine. If ovulation does not occur, the dosage is doubled, tripled, or quadrupled. Occasionally, there is overstimulation of the ovary, resulting in multiple births. This is probably the reason why this product is often called the fertility pill.

3. Pergonal is used when clomiphene citrate does not produce ovulation. Pergonal is FSH extracted from the urine of postmenopausal women. This is a very elaborate process and the drug is therefore very expensive.

4. Bromocriptine is a drug that can be used when ovulation is inhibited by excess amounts of prolactin, a pituitary hormone that stimulates the breast to produce milk. Bromocriptine suppresses prolactin and thus helps induce ovulation. The elevated prolactin level may be due to a tumor in the pituitary gland, a problem that needs to be resolved as it may represent a greater medical problem.

If the Fallopian tubes are blocked because of a previous tubal ligation, or from a stricture following an infection, it may be possible to unblock the system with microsurgery. In general, reversal of a tubal ligation is less successful than reversal of a vasectomy. Infectious strictures are even more difficult to reverse. Often, rather than attempt to unblock the tubes, in vitro fertilization (test-tube baby) is considered.

Endometriosis

A large number of infertile women have a disease called endometriosis. It may account for twenty percent of cases of female infertility.

Endometriosis is a peculiar condition in which tissue that normally lines the uterus is found elsewhere. The most frequent sites are the ovaries and peritoneal coverings of pelvic organs, such as the Fallopian tubes and uterine ligaments, but it can be found in many other locations, such as the rectal wall, bladder wall, ureter, etc. This tissue behaves like uterine tissue, bleeding periodically, and because it cannot drain out when it is located outside the uterine lining, it can promote scarring. One theory holds that endometriosis is due to a backflow of menstrual blood through the tubes and into the abdominal cavity. I have seen endometriosis involving the lining of the bladder. It is difficult to explain how uterine lining can find its way into the bladder, which raises questions about the theory. Furthermore, endometriosis has been found in the lung, limb muscles, and bones.

Endometriosis is associated with painful menstruation and infertility. The condition is now treated with a drug called danazol. This blocks FSH and LH production from the pituitary gland and, in effect, produces a temporary menopause. The treatment is continued for about six months and is then discontinued. Menstruation returns after about a month or so, and in more than half the cases of endometriosis, fertility is restored.

ARTIFICIAL INSEMINATION Artificial insemination takes place when the ejaculate is delivered to the vagina by means other than that of the penis. The semen can come from the husband or from an anonymous donor.

If the husband has a low sperm count, it would seem logical to suggest storing his semen, perhaps concentrating it, and using it at the most appropriate moment. To date, however, all attempts to improve the quality of the sperm outside the body have not proven successful. At some hospitals, doctors have tried squirting relatively poor-quality ejaculate directly into the uterus, bypassing the mucus at the cervix, which may be acting as a plug. The merit of this procedure has not yet been established.

Anonymous donor artificial insemination is another story. Undoubtedly, it works. Most hospitals report pregnancy at a rate of one in four attempts. The ethics and the morality underlying the procedure remain clouded. Doctors involved with anonymous donor insemination feel that the total number of cases around the world obviates medical-legal concerns.

The facts are as follows: the husband has an irreversible infertility problem; the wife is normal. The couple face a number of options. They might choose to accept their fate. They might give their name to an adoption agency. They might consider anonymous donor artificial insemination. For many, it is not an easy choice to make.

I have encountered husbands who were for artificial insemination while their wives were not. Sometimes, the wives are for it, and the husbands are not. One husband wanted to terminate the marriage and allow his wife a chance at "fulfillment." The tearful wife would hear none of it. Another wife could not understand why her husband would not accept the idea of the anonymous donor. Sometimes, the couple will try to trick me into taking sides. No matter what the final decision, the question rankles, and it is certainly not an easy decision to make.

Once the decision is made to proceed, further questions are raised. How successful is the procedure? One in four, as a rule. Any chance of malformations? Yes, but no more than the population at large. In fact, according to reports, it is less. Who are the donors? Medical students, by and large; occasionally, other university students. How carefully will the donor be matched with the husband? Race, color, and religion are currently possible. Do you foresee any long-term problems? Only the chance of consanguinity. What do you mean? That the child will grow up and marry a close relative (currently an extremely remote chance). Any other problems? There is a growing tendency among adopted children to search for their biological parents. Perhaps children who are products of anonymous semen may seek their biological father. What's my answer to that? I don't have any. What about the chances of catching AIDS? If the donor has AIDS and is unconscionable enough to serve as a donor, AIDS can be transmitted, as has already occurred. The chances of an AIDS transmission, however, are extremely remote.

The actual process of insemination is no more complicated than a routine pelvic examination. A speculum (what the gynecologist uses to examine the cervix and do a Pap smear) is placed inside the woman's vagina, and the semen, which is in a syringe, is simply squirted against the cervix. Occasionally, if there is a problem with conception, the gynecologist may use clomiphene citrate to stimulate ovulation so that the insemination can be timed for a convenient date.

THE TEST-TUBE BABY Dr. Robert Edwards and Dr. Patrick Steptoe startled the scientific world when they announced that a little girl born in England during the summer of 1978 had been conceived in a test tube. The mother had Fallopian tubes that were damaged beyond repair, but in every other way the parents were normal.

Test-tube babies are produced by a fine-tuning of science and nature. Doctors use a laparoscope (an instrument like a cystoscope, but which is surgically inserted into the abdominal cavity just under the umbilicus to see and manipulate inside the abdominal cavity) to obtain eggs from the ovary of the mother. The monthly release of the egg from the ovary can be timed exactly. Before it occurs, the ovary produces more and more estrogen which is monitored by examining the estrogen in the urine. Just before ovulation, there is a sudden increase in the level of LH and the woman is prepared for the laparoscopy.

When the ovary is examined at just this moment, there are a few dark bubbles on the surface. By using the laparoscope as a guide, a tiny, long needle is passed through the abdominal wall and into the bubble, suctioning out the fluid containing the egg. Normally, the bubble would have burst and the released egg would be captured by the free end of the Fallopian tube.

Sperm incubated in a special solution are then mixed with the egg. Different laboratories are reporting that no more than 35,000 sperm may be necessary for fertilization to occur under these conditions. It should be stated, however, that 35,000 sperm from a fertile donor may be different from 35,000 sperm from an infertile donor. Nevertheless, the creation of test-tube babies from men with low sperm counts becomes a possibility. At this time, most laboratories are hesitant to embark on this experiment because it is costly and less likely to be successful than when there is a normal sperm count.

The penetration of the sperm into the egg can be examined under the microscope. The nutrients are then changed and, at the eight-cell stage, the embryo is placed inside the uterus.

The entire process is extraordinarily simple, and extraordinarily complex. The pioneering efforts of Edwards and Steptoe have been duplicated by many laboratories around the world. Almost every medical center will attest to a long trial-and-error period and, even today, the process is in no way routine.

Furthermore, the concept of test-tube babies has opened up other possibilities. For example, the eight-cell embryos can be frozen and kept indefinitely. Not all embryos survive the freezing and thawing, but many do. It is also possible to use a surrogate mother, perhaps because the natural mother has lost her uterus or cannot tolerate a normal pregnancy. (Or the mother may have lost her ovaries, but has a normal uterus.) Might she then not "borrow" an egg, have it fertilized by her husband's sperm, and have the embryo implanted into her uterus?

The moral, ethical, political, and religious quagmire created by legitimate scientific research staggers the imagination. I feel that our ethicists, lawyers, doctors, and politicians would be foolish to draw rigid rules, for what is right in one circumstance will be wrong in another. And the moral issues are not confined to the outer reaches of medical practice. I face them, for example, when a young man is referred to me for a premarital fertility assessment.

"Why do you want a sperm count?" I ask.

"My fiancée and I feel it would be nice to know."

"Do you realize that the test cannot tell you if you will be a father or not?"

"How so?"

"You may have a normal sperm count, but that does not guarantee a pregnancy. Worse, you may have a relatively low count: I report it to you and you might develop a potential problem that might never have occurred had the test never been done."

"You think I should not have a sperm test?"

"I don't advise it. React to a medical problem, don't create one."

As somebody has said: "Don't fix what ain't broken."

The advice seems to satisfy some patients. Others will insist on having the tests done. Do I then give in, or do I tell them to find someone else to order it? I am not sure I have resolved the dilemma in my own mind.

Why does it take millions of sperm to create a pregnancy; I thought it took only one?

Thousands or hundreds of thousands of sperm must bombard and eat through the wall of the egg before one sperm can actually penetrate. Research is being done on how the egg wall can be digested by other means, so that pregnancy may occur with fewer sperm. We do not know if tampering with the process whereby the wall of the egg is prepared for the penetration will create more deformed offspring or not.

My wife and I have children from our previous marriages. Why do we have an infertility problem now?

It may be simply that you are now older and the chances of conception decline with age in both men and women.

Since my problem is a low sperm count, why can't you store and then concentrate the sperm?

I don't think that this question has been seriously examined by research scientists. On the one hand, several ejaculates of normal sperm are regularly frozen, stored, and used at a later date without significant loss of fertility. On the other hand, attempts to store, then concentrate several sperm collections appear to result in a substantial loss of viable sperm. Somehow, the two stories do not quite correspond. It should provide a fertile area for research.

When there is wide variation in the sperm count, is it a reflection of the person or the laboratory?

Lab errors can play a role, but the more likely source of the fluctuating count is the patient. We do not know why this occurs.

Why can't you use my sperm, even if it has a low count, and fertilize my wife's egg in a test tube?

There is no reason why this cannot be tried. Most doctors, however, want to restrict the technique to women with blocked Fallopian tubes, since there is a successful track record for this problem. It has not yet been established that test-tube fertilization can occur with a low sperm count ejaculate.

If my wife and I were less anxious, would our fertility problem get better?
The evidence that this is so is largely anecdotal. Stories of couples who became parents when they finally gave up on the idea of ever becoming parents are told again and again. What is not often related are stories of the many couples who remain childless after they give up.

Is it possible for a person to be born with testicles but without sperm ducts (vas deferens)? Can anything be done about it?
The vas deferens can be absent on one side or both sides. At the present time, we have no way of substituting for, or creating, a sperm duct.

Can a testicle produce male hormones if it can't produce sperm?
Yes. The male hormone is produced by Leydig's cells, within the testicle. These cells are quite hardy. Sperm, on the other hand, are produced when cells, lining a coiled and twisted tubule, are transformed from stationary cells into mobile, tadpole-like units. The sperm-producing process is fragile, and the mechanism easily injured.

Are children born to couples with infertility problems likely to have birth abnormalities?
There is no scientific evidence to support this fear. Indeed, the clinical impression is that miscarriages may be more frequent, but birth defects are less common.

6 VASECTOMY AND REVERSAL

ETHICS AND MORALITY **H**omo sapiens are very sexual creatures. No other animal delights in sexual intercourse the way we do. We respect no season, no time of day, no preordained frequency. I do not believe all of Freud's doctrines, but I do think he was right in suggesting sex as a driving force in the behavior of man. But how are we to cope with the ethical and moral repercussions? Should respect for the sanctity of life be extended to every living sperm in the ejaculate? If not, why not? Should we respect the sanctity of the fertilized egg or embryo, or only when the fetus is capable of life outside the uterus? And who can claim authority to make these decisions?

I have no quarrel with patients and doctors who feel that sterilization contravenes their religious principles. I object only when and if they feel they must impose their convictions on others. Theirs is an arbitrary morality. This was clear to me when a blind man, already a father of two children, came to me because his parish priest had objected to his considering a vasectomy. I referred him to a younger priest, who approved his request for a vasectomy without hesitation.

My only qualms about a vasectomy occur when a young man requests it. Often he is unmarried but certain that he should not bring any children into this "ugly" world. I will suggest that he reconsider, that a deep love might change his outlook. He is usually certain it will not. And if I will not consider it, he claims, he will simply find somebody who will. Is my conscience better served by refusing him, certain that he will be treated elsewhere? What I will do is delay the decision and suggest we meet again in a year's time. If the young man is then still certain he should have a vasectomy, he will have no further argument from me. Some young men have returned, a year later, and have had their operation. Some have not returned, and a few have come back to thank me for giving them the time to reconsider.

I have never done a sham vasectomy, as a colleague of mine once did. His patient's wife had become pregnant and the patient asked for a repeat vasectomy. A check of his ejaculate revealed no sperm. Rather than create a problem for "a nice couple," my friend elected to carry out a sham operation, cutting only the skin. He asked if I would have done the same. I said I would not have, but I did not face this problem.

Normally, I have no moral qualms about vasectomy. We do need some form of birth control. And in a stable domestic situation, when the family has been completed, vasectomy is the most reliable and least traumatic means.

THE OPERATION Male sterilization or vasectomy is the simplest "cutting" operation I do. I have carried out the procedure thousands of times in my office, and not once has a patient required hospitalization due to a complication. My secretary allots me twenty minutes for each case. This includes the time to answer questions, allow the patient to undress and dress, disinfect the skin, and occasionally to shave the upper scrotum when the patient has forgotten to come prepared as directed. Thus the actual time for surgery is closer to ten minutes.

At a refresher course for family physicians some years ago, I suggested that vasectomy can be carried out without losing a drop of blood (certainly less than five drops), and without the use of stitches inside or outside. Two doctors in the audience were incredulous and asked if they could witness me at work. I told them they were welcome if my patients did not object. I can't recall now how well it went, whether they saw one procedure or two, but I know that the surgical trauma was as minimal as I had described it to them.

My technique for vasectomy is as follows: First, I disinfect the scrotum with iodine solution. Then I locate one of the vas and keep it fixed under the skin between my index finger and thumb. With my other hand I inject a local anesthetic into the scrotum near my

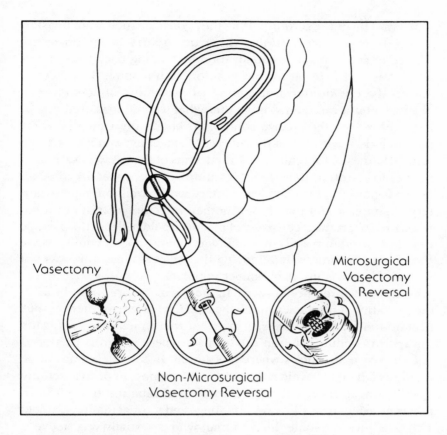

Vasectomy

Microsurgical
Vasectomy
Reversal

Non-Microsurgical
Vasectomy Reversal

thumb tip, just on top of and on either side of the vas. I use one percent Xylocaine, injecting about two milliliters of the solution and raising what looks like a mosquito bite. There is very little pain if the fluid is injected very slowly. A three-millimeter cut is then made into the "mosquito bite." The anesthetic works instantaneously, so there is no delay. A toothed forceps grasps the vas, and then for the first time the hand localizing the vas is released. A clamp with a curved and pointed end, known as a towel clip, is then looped around the vas. The surrounding thick outer cover of the vas is teased away, a one-centimeter length of vas excised, and the cut ends burned with needle-tipped electrocautery. The procedure is then repeated on the other vas.

How much variation can there be for such a simple procedure? Surprisingly, quite a bit. Some doctors make a one- to two-inch cut in the middle of the scrotum. Why they consider such a big incision necessary is a mystery to me. Other doctors try to minimize the chance of spontaneous recanalization by looping back the cut end of the vas and fixing it in that position with a stitch. But there is always the one-in-four-or-five-hundred possibility of spontaneous reversal after a vasectomy, no matter what technique is used. Looping may reduce the chance somewhat, but in my view, the extra manipulation, with its increased risk of infection, is not worth the return. Some doctors cauterize the cut ends of the vas with saturated phenol (as is often done for the stumps of the appendix after an appendectomy). This chemical cautery works well, but electrocautery is simplest and thus best. Another vasectomy variation, notorious for a short time, consisted of placing a gold pellet in the passage of the vas. The supposed advantage was that the doctor could reverse the procedure simply by removing the pellet. In fact, this was not so and the procedure is no longer popular.

I test for the presence of sperm in the ejaculate three months after the operation. I used to examine the ejaculate after two months, but I found too many positive specimens at that time. Vasectomy cuts the sperm conduit between the testicles where sperm is produced and the seminal vesicles where it is stored. But the depot has to be totally evacuated to avoid conception. The number of postvasectomy ejaculations necessary to assure absolute evacuation has not been precisely calculated. Early reports suggested ten ejaculations; others suggested twenty, some thirty. A man who is sexually very active is likely to clear his depot more quickly than a man who is less active. In general, a younger man has a negative specimen before an older man. Three months, though, is an appropriate time for the first check. If there is no sperm in the ejaculate examined under the microscope at this time, a second specimen is tested. I send my patients to an independent lab for a third check. Even so, I warn my patients of the remote risk of spontaneous reversal and suggest a sperm test once a year.

I was sued once early in my career. After one sample that showed no sperm, the patient was advised to return for his second test. He thought better of it and returned only when his wife became pregnant. A sperm test then revealed copious numbers of sperm. He had had a spontaneous reversal. A second vasectomy was carried out without complications. Subsequently, I was served a subpoena. I went to court to make a formal statement, but fortunately the case was dropped. The surgical consent form now in use specifies that the procedure cannot be guaranteed.

OTHER METHODS
OF BIRTH CONTROL
Most other methods of contraception are unhealthy or less reliable when compared to a vasectomy.

In any given year, twenty-five percent of couples practicing the rhythm method of contraception are faced with an unwanted pregnancy.

Condoms and diaphragms, with or without spermicidal jelly, are only slightly more reliable, with undesired pregnancy occurring five to fifteen percent of the time.

The intrauterine device (IUD) is considered to be ninety-eight percent effective, but it has fallen into relative disfavor because of the risk of permanent infertility as well as the more immediate problems of pain, bleeding, and migration of the device. I know of one case where the IUD had migrated into the abdomen. Problems with the IUD are uncommon but are alarming enough to persuade most pharmaceutical firms to discontinue the product.

The contraceptive pill may make pragmatic sense. It is, after all, 99.9 percent effective, but it is so unsafe and unfair to women that I wonder why the women's movement has not made a bigger issue of it. When the pill was developed, it was tested on a vast number of female volunteers. It was then judged safe over many thousand menstrual cycles, implying that women could take the pill indefinitely. What was not clearly spelled out was that there was a difference between 5,000 women testing the pill for three cycles and 50 women testing it for a lifetime, even though the two groups represented comparable numbers of menstrual cycles. Clots in the veins, strokes, and death caused by the pill came as a total surprise to the medical profession fifteen to seventeen years after the pill was launched. It can be stated today that the pill was never properly tested over time. It is argued that since complications occur in less than 1 in 1,000 women on the pill, its use is justifiable. This may be so, except for the one woman who happens to be the unlucky statistic. Young women must decide whether the 1-per-1,000 chance of a clot in the deep vein with its risk of a potential fatal clot to the lungs, or the threefold increased risk of stroke, are worth it. The actual death rate attributable to the pill is 1.5 per 100,000 women between the age of twenty and thirty-five. Women not taking the pill have a death rate from blood clot in the lung or brain of 0.2 per 100,000. The pill increases the risk 7.5 times. Women over forty increase their chances of heart attacks 5 times by taking the pill. Thus most concerned physicians will not allow women over forty to take the pill, especially if they are overweight, smoke, have high blood pressure, or are diabetic. The risks are simply not acceptable.

Female sterilization, despite progress, is still a much more formidable undertaking than vasectomy. No matter what technique is employed, the peritoneal cavity has to be opened before the Fallopian tubes can be tied off. This means cutting through the front wall of the abdomen surgically or piercing the wall with a laparoscope to see inside the abdomen. The Fallopian tubes are clipped and the ends banded or electrocauterized. There is always the risk of infection, which can become peritonitis (pus collection inside the abdomen, as in a ruptured appendix). A tubal ligation can only be safely carried out in the operating room of a hospital and almost always under general anesthetic. And, just as with vasectomy, there is a 1-in-400-to-500 chance of a spontaneous reconnection.

WHAT CAN GO WRONG WITH VASECTOMY

Vasectomy may be a simple office procedure, but it is not free of complications.

There can be internal bleeding, turning the scrotum black, blue, hard, and painful. This can occur when there has been excessive probing and dissection by an inexperienced surgeon, or when the patient is too physically active in the first few days following the procedure. When bleeding occurs, it is not readily contained by the surrounding tissue and skin because the scrotal sac is loose tissue—and there is space for blood to collect. A pressure dressing or athletic support worn immediately after the operation may help, but the problem is best avoided by meticulous surgery and conservative postsurgical behavior: I instruct my patients to lie low for forty-eight hours after a vasectomy. They can walk, but not jog or run. On the few occasions that a black and blue scrotum has occurred, patients invariably confess that they did not follow instructions. They had so little discomfort that they thought they could chance playing hockey or football.

84

Another potential complication is wound infection, causing pain and fever. Internal bleeding and infection can occur together, usually reflecting poor surgical technique. Some doctors try to prevent infection by offering a course of antibiotics after the operation. This is not necessary and constitutes improper use of antibiotics. In the rare event when there is a wound infection, a broad spectrum antibiotic, such as tetracycline, is prescribed.

Perhaps an even greater surgical error is to confuse another tissue for the vas. I have heard a number of patients say that they have had an unsuccessful vasectomy. A second operation was necessary, they say, because of the possibility of a third vas. I have never seen a third vas and doubt that such a condition exists. It is a convenient excuse for the doctor. On the other hand, an absent vas on one or both sides is not so uncommon. This may be a rare complication of diethylstilbestrol (DES), a form of estrogen taken by the mother during pregnancy.

Finally, as discussed before, the cut, tied, or cauterized ends of the vas may come together and continuity of the passage be re-established in spontaneous recanalization. This can be due to improper surgical technique, but not necessarily. The possibility is one in four hundred or five hundred cases, and the risks are highest in the few months immediately after the operation, but can occur at any time. I advise my patients to have a sperm test once a year, but not many patients follow the advice.

Unfounded Complications of Vasectomy

Some of the early objections to vasectomy were made by people who were philosophically opposed to the operation and who sought scientific support for their stance. For example, it was suggested that seventy percent of men with vasectomies would develop arthritis. At first glance, the statistics were startling: seventy percent of vasectomized men did indeed develop arthritis. But seventy percent of the adult population normally develops arthritis anyway, and thus vasectomized males are not any more prone to arthritis. The operation itself does not play any contributory role.

Another investigator found that vasectomized rats lost interest in sex and that the male hormone level in the bloodstream of these rats dropped to castrate levels. So he issued a warning to the human male population. But when the vas is cut in rats, pressure builds up in the pipes behind the cut and the testicles are totally destroyed. In man, there is only a mild buildup of pressure and no damage to the testicles. This is one of the problems with animal research. Certain results obtained for one species are not transferable to another.

More recently, another reputable scientist found that vasectomy was associated with irrefutable evidence of accelerated atherosclerosis. Again, this was a finding peculiar to one species of monkeys and not substantiated in man.

At this point in time, it can be concluded that vasectomy in the fertile man is safe, simple, and effective.

VASECTOMY REVERSAL Although the patient and the doctor undertake a vasectomy as an irreversible procedure, personal circumstances do change and there may be a need to consider reversing the procedure. Sometimes the death of a wife or a child leads to a reconsideration, but the most common reason for reversal is the desire to have a child with a new partner. Sometimes the reasons are more bizarre. I remember one man whose Indian guru convinced him that he must be made "whole." The psychiatrist to whom I referred the patient supported the request, so I proceeded with the surgery.

Unlike a vasectomy, the reversal is most often an in-hospital procedure and there is considerable controversy among specialists about which technique to use. Imagine joining two spools of thread head to head and aligning the hole and you have visualized the surgical challenge of a vasectomy reversal. One school of experts firmly believes that microsurgical connections are essential for success, while another feels that the use of the microscope is overrated. I have done the procedure both with and without a microscope. When the microscope is used, the procedure tends to be more tedious and time-consuming. It is also exhausting. But there is an enormous sense of accomplishment at the end of the procedure. Using the microscope, several tiny stitches join the inner walls of each cut end and several larger stitches bring the thick outer walls together. When the microscope is not used, approximately four stitches that traverse the entire thick wall of the vas are used to bring the ends together. It seems to me that the results in both procedures are comparable and that the arguments about technique simply shift the emphasis away from the real issue: how to test for the results.

There is no safe method to test the surgical repair. Fluids or dyes cannot be injected at one end to exit from the other. The presence of sperm implies a successful operation, but the quantity and quality of the sperm do not reflect the quality of the surgery performed. A high count does not necessarily mean a better sewing job, an inferior count does not mean poor surgery. There are other factors to contend with, such as the expectation that higher counts occur when the interval between the vasectomy and the reversal is under five years. Then again, although this expectation is firmly entrenched in the medical literature, some of the highest sperm counts I have seen after a reversal occurred after intervals of ten to fifteen years. Thus the only important measure of success is a pregnancy. But hospitals that report ninety percent pregnancy rates cannot prove that they have eliminated the "milkman" factor. Testing for paternity is theoretically possible, but does not seem appropriate in most circumstances.

Patients who request a vasectomy reversal are told that the success rate ranges from fifty to ninety percent. I suspect the first figure is more accurate than the second.

Vasectomies and vasectomy reversals can present complications for the doctor as well. Once, six months after I had reversed a vasectomy, a patient returned to tell me that his wife was pregnant. I congratulated him but expressed surprise. Normally, I suggested, I don't bother to check the sperm count until nine to twelve months after the reversal because the results before that are usually disappointing. But if the wife was pregnant and everybody was happy, why not rejoice?

Three months later, my patient returned to tell me that his wife had left him and had taken the baby. He said that he recalled my implying that the baby might not be his, and that if such were the case, he was determined to terminate support for her. "Can you do some tests?" he asked.

I suggested that we do a sperm count. If the operation had not been successful, we would have laboratory evidence that he was not the father. The semen analysis showed more than a hundred million very motile sperm per milliliter—he was quite fertile. I imagined countless uncomfortable days in court.

But the patient returned to tell me not to worry. His former wife confessed that he was not the father and that she would seek no support. There would be no lawsuits. Could he be considered for another vasectomy? he asked. I politely ushered him to the door. . . .

QUESTIONS AND ANSWERS

Where does the sperm go after a vasectomy?
Sperm live out their normal life span, die, disintegrate, and within hours cruising white blood cells swallow up the remains. There is no buildup of pressure, no extra discomfort, and no danger.

Do you have to shave my scrotum to do a vasectomy?
The cut is made into the hair-bearing portion of the upper scrotum. Unshaven, the hair is likely to obstruct the operation or find its way into the wound, like an ingrown toenail. What is less certain, today, is whether shaving reduces the risk of wound infection. Indeed, a number of studies suggest that shaving the abdomen is associated with an increased rate of infection in the skin wound.

I ask my patients to come with the upper one-inch-square of the scrotum shaved on each side.

Will I need antibiotics or painkillers after the vasectomy?
Antibiotics are unnecessary. On the rare occasion when an abscess forms, the pus should be cultured and an appropriate antibiotic prescribed. Strong narcotics are also unnecessary. A mild painkiller, such as acetaminophen (Tylenol), may be used. Ice packs applied to the scrotum are probably the most effective method of controlling discomfort. Ice packs are easily made by placing ice cubes in a plastic bag and then covering the bag with a towel.

Can I get right back to normal afterward?
If there is bleeding from the tiny veins that surround the vas during the operation, it is controlled by electrocautery. If the patient is too active afterward, bleeding can restart at the points of cautery. Since this is better avoided than treated, it is best to keep a low profile for a few days.

How soon after can I have sexual intercourse?

Wait two days, and then use your common sense. Hold off if there is any discomfort; but if there is no discomfort, it is up to you. Of course, until the ejaculate is clear of sperm, contraceptive precautions must be taken.

Will the vasectomy affect my virility or my potency?

Virility and potency are largely a reflection of the male hormone (testosterone) level. Neither the production of the hormone, nor its release into the bloodstream, is altered by a vasectomy.

What about delayed complications of vasectomy, such as cancer?

More than a generation (twenty-five years) has passed, and millions of vasectomies have been performed throughout the world. Even in this large sample, no worrisome later complications have been recorded.

How soon after a vasectomy reversal can I become a father?

Theoretically, the first live sperm can appear three months after a reversal. In fact, live sperm in large numbers are seldom seen until a year later. I have seen counts that were low a year after reversal improve with the years. I have also seen high counts worsen over the years.

Is it possible that too much of the vas can be removed, making a reversal impossible?

Gaps of five centimeters and more can be bridged. But with a large gap, it takes more cutting of surrounding tissue before the two ends can be brought together, and the surgical trauma is greater. A vasectomy done close to the testicle is less likely to be successfully reversed than a vasectomy done a few centimeters away. This is because when the cut is near the epididymis, the far end of the vas must be connected to a tiny tubule within the epididymis, rather than to the other end of the vas. This microsurgery is less likely to be successful.

Why does vasectomy reversal not always work?
There are a number of explanations. The technique may have been faulty, or the testicles may not recover their capacity to produce sperm, or, if they recover, they may do so with less vigor. We do not know why certain testicles are unable to recover or what percentage of men will have this problem.

7 SCROTAL LUMPS

Back in the fifteenth, sixteenth, and seventeenth centuries, it was popular for men to wear what is called a codpiece. This was an ornamented, fortified bag, or flap, with a concealed opening, attached to the front of men's close-fitting breeches. It was designed to make men look larger than they were.

In our own day, we have certain rock stars and pop singers padding their groins to enhance image and appeal. And in my own practice I have had a number of patients who decided not to remove lumps that had developed in their scrotum because they wanted to look like "supermen."

I remember one man who had a lump the size of an egg in his scrotum. When assured that the fluid-filled lump was not cancerous and could not become cancerous, he happily announced that he would pass it off as a third testicle. He'd already had considerable success with the ladies, he confessed. He'd just come to me to make sure he wasn't sitting on a cancer.

It was wise of him to see a doctor because lumps in the scrotum are sometimes benign and sometimes cancerous.

This is a chapter about scrotal lumps—something you might never know existed, even if you had them. They may cause no pain and, even when squeezed, may cause no distress.

Cancer of the testicle is the one dangerous lump. It is also one of the lumps that can be painless and nontender. The following chapter will explain how you can examine yourself for this disease. Self-examination for testicular cancer should be carried out at regular intervals by all men in the same way all women should examine themselves for breast lumps.

Almost all the other lumps within the scrotum are less ominous. Let us begin with the benign lumps. Innocent lumps include: hernia, hydrocele, varicocele, spermatocele, cyst of epididymis, epididymitis, and mumps orchitis. Among all these benign scrotal lumps, there are two—the hernia and the hydrocele—that can reach enormous proportions.

HERNIA A hernia is a protrusion of an organ or part of an organ through a wall of the cavity in which it is normally contained. It usually occurs because of a combination of inborn weakness and straining. The straining may be due to lifting heavy objects, straining to urinate when there is an obstruction such as an enlarged prostate, or straining to defecate when constipated. The hernia is generally described in relation to its site or origin. Thus there is a diaphragmatic hernia (hiatus hernia), which is the protrusion of the stomach upward into the chest cavity; an umbilical hernia, in which the intestine or part of an intestine protrudes at the belly button; a ventral hernia, where a weakness in the anterior abdominal wall, usually after closure of a surgical opening of the abdomen, allows intestines to protrude; and inguinal hernias, of which there are three varieties.

A protrusion of intestine at the groin because of a weak front wall is called a direct inguinal hernia; a protrusion of the gut into the lower leg beside where the vessel pulsation can be felt is called a femoral hernia; and a protrusion of intestine through the passage taken by the testicle to reach the scrotum is called an indirect inguinal hernia. The indirect inguinal hernia is the one that can reach the size of a football.

A hernia is called "reducible" if the intestine can be pushed back into the abdomen, "incarcerated" if it cannot be pushed back, and "strangulated" if the blood flow to the intestine is cut off. This happens when the ringlike opening of the peritoneal tube chokes the bowel.

Some patients may choose to live with a hernia if there is no distress. Others may purchase a truss, which is a padded belt that works like the thumb in the dike, plugging the site where the hernia starts. The only cure for a hernia is surgical repair—which is mandatory when there is strangulation.

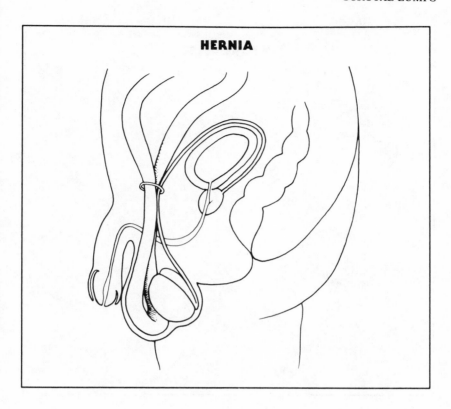

HERNIA

The hernia repair consists of pushing the intestine back into the cavity where it belongs, cutting off the hernia sac, which is the tonguelike protrusion of the abdominal wall lining, and repairing the opening and weakness in the wall that gave rise to the hernia. There are a number of techniques that have been evolved to effect the repair. In principle, strong ligamentous tissues are sewn to solid tissues, like the lining of bone. When naturally occurring supporting tissue is unavailable, a synthetic material, like a Dacron mesh, is used to create the support.

Most men have had the "cough test" done to detect an early hernia. The doctor pushes up the scrotal skin toward the abdomen. He asks the patient to cough and feels for a bulge against his finger. If there's a bulge, an early hernia has been detected.

93

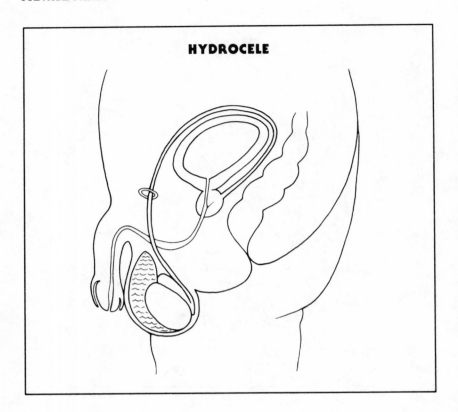

HYDROCELE

HYDROCELE If the peritoneal tube associated with the formation of a hernia is closed at the top but filled with fluid near the testicle, it is a hydrocele. To detect a hydrocele, the doctor takes his patient into a dark room and places a lighted flashlight directly up against the scrotum. If there is a hydrocele in the scrotum, the fluid in it will show up as a red glow. The potential for hydrocele formation exists in every man. An injury to the scrotum or an irritation to the testicle can stimulate secretion of fluid from the cells that make up the peritoneal tube. Such fluid will not disappear on its own. If the hydrocele is not large and not causing distress, it can be left alone. When the collection of fluid is excessive (I have drained as much as two quarts), there can be discomfort, even pain. The pale, clear yellow fluid can be removed with a needle. If the hydrocele is due to an injury, the fluid will not reaccumulate.

But the cause of most hydroceles is unknown, and the fluid of most of them reaccumulates since the causal factors remain. If after the fluid is removed, a sclerosing chemical is instilled, further reaccumulation can often be avoided. A commonly instilled chemical is the antibiotic tetracycline. Instillation of 250 milligrams of the drug dissolved in about two milliliters of a local anesthetic is often, but not always, successful.

Surgery for a hydrocele is very simple: the bulk of the hydrocele sac (peritoneal tube) is cut away, and what remains is turned inside out. As a result, the fluid-secreting surface is now in contact with the inner skin of the scrotum, rather than that of the testicle with which it made previous contact. The scrotal tissue blots up any fluid that is secreted, unlike the testicular tissue which cannot absorb fluid. An operation for a hydrocele can be undertaken on an outpatient basis, but it is more common to be hospitalized for a day or two.

Surgery for a hydrocele is undertaken if the patient is uncomfortable with the size of the fluid collection. He may find it heavy, uncomfortable, or embarrassing if it shows through his trousers. Usually at this stage, it is the size of a large orange. Some men, however, are not overly concerned by their hydrocele and live comfortably with it.

VARICOCELE   A varicocele is another benign lump that can occur in the scrotum. It is, simply, a collection of distended veins. Veins are part of the circulatory system that takes blood back to the heart. There is no pump in the venous system that generates pressure such as the heart muscle does in the arterial system. The venous system is a low-pressure system that depends on pressure from adjacent tissue, gravity, and the arrival of more blood to push the flow. Its flow toward the heart is prevented from going backward by a system of one-way flap valves. (You can demonstrate the presence of these valves in your own body by letting your arm dangle until the surface veins are filled with blood. Then, with your finger, milk the blood out of one vein, down toward your fingertip. Blood will refill the vein only to the point of the one-way valve.)

However, the veins draining blood from the left testicle are particularly vulnerable to being overfilled. This is because the testicular vein empties far away (one and a half to two feet) and, also, at a

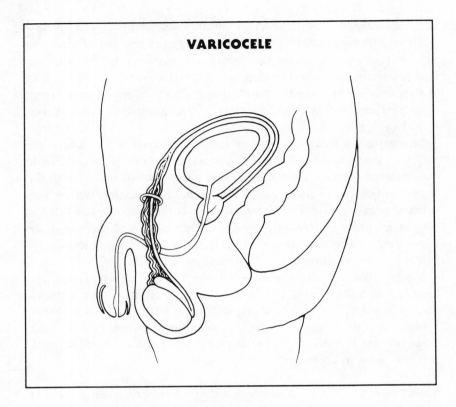

VARICOCELE

right angle into the next vein. At least one percent of the male population have a left-sided varicocele. The right side is less vulnerable because the right testicular vein drains lower down, and obliquely, into a larger vein.

It is simple to diagnose a varicocele. It feels as if there is a tangle of worms in the scrotum. This is so because it is not one vein but a cluster of veins that has become distended.

The presence of a varicocele does not necessarily indicate a need for surgery. A varicocele may be symptom-free, or the cause of a vague discomfort. Surgical correction is considered only when there is considerable discomfort, or when there is an infertility problem with a low sperm count. (This is discussed further in the chapter on infertility.)

SPERMATOCELE,
CYST OF EPIDIDYMIS

A spermatocele is a fluid-filled lump that arises from the epididymis. Most men feel it as a lump in their scrotum, which they often confuse with cancer, although the spermatocele is absolutely benign. How and why it occurs is not known. The epididymis is a conglomeration of tiny tubules directly behind the testicle into which the sperm empty en route to the vas deferens. When a tubule blows up, and fills with a milky fluid, often containing sperm, it is a spermatocele. The spherical lump can be as small as a pea, the size of a golf ball, or even larger. This blowout of a tubule need not totally block the passage of sperm, and even if it does, fertility is unaffected because of the other side. No noticeable change will be detected in the ejaculate because so little of the total volume of ejaculate comes from the epididymis.

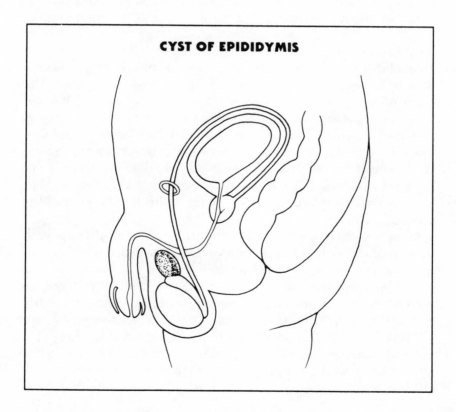

CYST OF EPIDIDYMIS

A similar fluid-filled lump in about the same location behind and above the testicle can be filled with clear colorless fluid. This is a cyst of the epididymis. Without examination of the fluid, the distinction between a spermatocele and a cyst of the epididymis cannot be made.

Spermatoceles and cysts of the epididymis can be left alone unless there is discomfort because they have grown uncomfortably large. Surgery is a simple matter requiring, at most, one day of hospitalization. The lump is approached directly through the scrotal skin and dissected off. Often, it can be removed as an intact sphere.

INFLAMMATORY SWELLING There are three reasons why the contents of the scrotum swell due to inflammation: (1) bacterial infection (epididymitis), (2) viral infection (mumps orchitis), (3) twisting of the testicle (torsion).

Epididymitis

An epididymitis is an infection of the epididymis, the tiny structure behind the testicle into which the sperm exit from the testicle. The infecting microorganism is most often a bowel bacteria, but the invading organism can also be chlamydia (a tiny bacteria that is transmitted sexually), a tubercle bacillus (which causes tuberculosis), skin bacteria, or a virus. The microorganisms enter the epididymis from the bloodstream or from the vas deferens. We do not know why bacteria in the bloodstream settle in the epididymis, but bacteria from the vas often flow back from infection in the bladder, prostate, or urethra.

An attack of epididymitis can vary from a benign swelling with some tenderness to a febrile illness that is incapacitating. A mild case may clear up with oral antibiotics. A severe case of epididymitis may extend into the testicle, causing it to swell and fill with pus. In a severe case, it is necessary to administer intravenous antibiotics and intravenous fluids. Bed rest, elevation of the scrotum, and application of ice packs are all part of the regime. Not too long ago, surgical drainage was carried out in severe cases, but today treatment using powerful antibiotics resolves the infection in most cases, and surgical drainage is seldom necessary.

98

Mumps Orchitis

Mumps is usually a childhood illness which attacks the parotid gland in front of the ear. When the infection occurs after puberty, there is a one-in-four chance of mumps occurring in the testicle (and in the ovary of females). When the disease attacks the testicle, it causes a painful swelling so that the testicle may appear to be five times its normal size. Sometimes the pain is so severe a doctor may freeze the nerve with an injection of a local anesthetic. Eventually, the swelling subsides and leaves the organ a shrunken shadow of itself, the size of a marble, useless as a sperm producer and questionable as a hormone producer. Fortunately, the virus usually attacks only one side.

Torsion

Torsion is a problem that occurs almost exclusively in adolescent boys. It is not impossible, however, for the problem to occur in older boys or grown men. In fact, it is a wonder that torsion does not occur more often. As has been described, the testicle drops into the scrotum like a yo-yo on its string. The string or "cord" contains blood vessels and a drainage tube (vas deferens) and it is wrapped in a spiraling muscle. When this muscle suddenly contracts (during sexual excitement or when physically injured), the testicle may twist within the scrotum. If a doctor can see a patient in this situation promptly, he will check to see if the epididymis is outside its normal posterior position. If it is, the doctor can usually untwist the testicle manually and put it back in its normal position. But if the patient waits, it will be only a matter of hours before the tissue swells with fluid. The anatomical landmarks become obscured and make simple detorsion impossible. Surgery is often necessary to untwist the torsion. After five to six hours of torsion, the testicle is unsalvageable and is removed.

It is often difficult to distinguish between a torsion and an epididymitis. Lifting the scrotum is supposed to lighten the pain of an epididymitis and worsen the pain of a torsion, but it is unsafe to rely on such a test. Thus when there is a chance that the problem might be a torsion, the patient is better off being taken to the operating room. I have seen at least half a dozen missed torsions in my career. One such case was a medical student, and the diagnosis was missed by my professor. Sometimes, surgery is carried out even

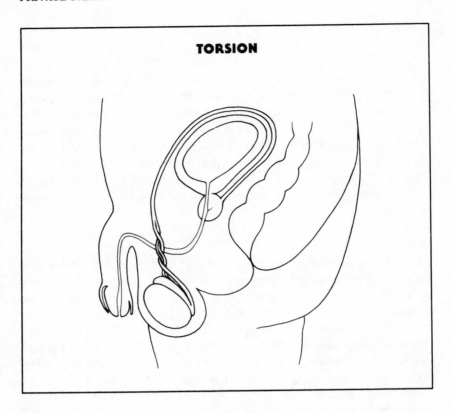

TORSION

though more than six hours have passed. The testicle is untwisted, bathed in warm salt solution, and watched for several minutes. If there is any sign of life in the organ, a little pink hue, it is left in. At the same time, or at a subsequent date, the opposite side is fixed with three stitches so that it cannot twist.

CANCER OF THE TESTICLE In men between the ages of twenty and forty, cancer of the testicle is the third leading cause of death and the most common cause of death due to a cancer in the western world. Three new cases per hundred thousand men are diagnosed every year.

It is prudent, therefore, for young men to learn to examine themselves for this cancer. The testicle should feel as smooth and firm as a hard-boiled egg without its shell. Almost the entire surface of the testicle, except for a small area in the back where the epididymis

100

attaches to it, can be examined through the thin scrotal skin. The examination is best accomplished in a warm bath or under the shower, with the testicle between the thumb and fingertips. A light touch with the fingertip is all that is necessary since the testicle is delicate and sensitive, and any undue pressure applied to it will cause nauseating pain. An irregularity of the surface, or a firm lump within the organ, should be regarded with suspicion. (An irregular surface and hardness can also be due to chronic infection.) If there is any question of a possible abnormality, it should be checked by a physician.

An early cancer has no symptoms. Even when a tumor has totally replaced the testicle, there may be no symptoms. On the other hand, a late cancer may be felt as a weight or a pulling sensation. Pain, caused by a bleeding into the tumor, or a blockage of the blood flow within the testicle, may also be an indication of cancer.

An ultrasound examination is a very sensitive, reliable test to assess the state of the testicle. The pattern of the sound waves bounced off the testicle is altered by a growth of no more than a millimeter in size. Ultrasound is more precise than a manual examination.

Cancer and the Undescended Testicle
The ultrasound test is particularly useful in men who have had surgery to bring down a testicle. Men born with an undescended testicle have a greater chance of getting testicular cancer than the normal population—their risk is twenty times higher. (Seven percent of the men who develop cancer of the testicle are born with an undescended testicle, and twenty percent of the time the cancer develops in the opposite, "normal" testicle.) Routine examination of this group of young men is often difficult because the surgery to bring down the testicle may have created anatomical distortions. Ultrasound helps make the necessary diagnosis.

Classification of Cancer of the Testicle
Cancer of the testicle is classified as germinal (arising from cells that produce sperm) or nongerminal (arising from any other cells). The nongerminal cancers are exceedingly rare and will, therefore, not be described.

Germinal tumors are categorized according to four different cell types:

101

1. Seminoma
2. Embryonal cell carcinoma
3. Teratocarcinoma
4. Choriocarcinoma

These four cell types can occur in pure form or in various combinations. When the tumor is pure, seminoma has the best prognosis. The prognosis for teratocarcinoma and embryonal cell carcinoma is better than the prognosis for choriocarcinoma. Long ago, a doctor observed that when there is an element of seminoma in a mixed tumor, the outlook improves; when there is an element of choriocarcinoma, the prognosis is poorer.

Eighty-five percent of teratocarcinoma and embryonal cell cancers secrete measurable chemicals into the bloodstream (alpha-feto-protein or beta-HCG). These two "markers" are used to follow the progress of the disease and to assess the patient's response to different treatments.

Choriocarcinoma also secretes a specific hormone (the beta subunit of human chorionic gonadotropin—beta-HCG). The levels of this hormone can be measured and used to monitor the progressive stages of this disease.

On occasion, pure seminoma can also secrete these "markers," but we don't know why this occurs irregularly.

Stage

Staging the tumor means defining the extent of the disease at the time of diagnosis. Testicular cancer is staged as follows:

STAGE A.   The tumor is confined to the testicle.

STAGE B1.   The tumor has spread to the lymph nodes, but less than five nodes are involved and none are larger than two centimeters.

STAGE B2.   More than five nodes are involved or there is evidence of a node larger than two centimeters.

STAGE B3.   The lymph nodes are massive and can probably be detected by a manual examination of the abdomen, but there is no apparent spread above the diaphragm.

STAGE C.   The cancer is above the diaphragm, or involves liver, lung, bone, or brain tissue.

Management

When testicular cancer is diagnosed, blood is immediately drawn for the markers and the patient is prepared for surgery. The testicle is removed through a groin incision similar to that used for a hernia repair. The testicle is simply pulled out of the scrotal sac by its cord. Radical removal is an exceedingly simple operation to perform.

While the pathologist studies the specimen, the patient is staged. A liver and bone scan, a lymphangiogram, and a CT scan are required to stage the disease. (Liver and bone scans are discussed in the section on prostate cancer.) A lymphangiogram is an X-ray technique which identifies the size, number, and position of the lymph nodes. It is done with two dyes. First, a dark dye, injected between the patient's toes, shows up the lymphatic channels as a dark streak under the skin. A lymphatic channel can then be dissected free, threaded with a tiny plastic tube, and injected with another dye that shows up on X ray. Subsequent X rays show the size and distribution of the lymph nodes. The CT scan, a computer-assisted X ray, reveals lymph nodes which are larger than two centimeters.

A seminoma can almost always be cured with surgical removal of the testicle and radiotherapy applied to the area under the diaphragm (which is the site of lymph-node drainage for the testicle). Radiotherapy is selected for this cancer because the gamma rays beamed directly to the cancer site are effective in destroying the cancer cells. When the seminoma has spread to areas above the diaphragm, and the disease is extensive, chemotherapy is often used as well. The reason chemotherapy is selected for cancer above the diaphragm is that radiotherapy would damage delicate lung tissue. Chemotherapy, injected in the vein in this situation, has a more generalized and beneficial effect on this cancer.

Teratocarcinoma and embryonal cell carcinoma often require lymph-node dissection to stage the disease. But if there is no evidence of cancer beyond the testicle, lymph-node dissection may be deferred. It is, however, necessary to follow up with CT scans and ultrasound examinations. It must be understood that if ever or whenever there is evidence of lymph node disease, chemotherapy must be started. If tests have already indicated that the disease has spread or that the lymph nodes are larger than two centimeters, lymph-node dissection is also unnecessary, since chemotherapy is started right away. Chemotherapy is an exhausting and trying ordeal and cannot be undertaken as a preventative measure.

Choriocarcinoma can be monitored by testing for the presence of gonadotropin. In positive cases, chemotherapy is necessary and often succeeds in controlling what used to be a uniformly fatal disease.

Cancer in young people is totally devastating, and as cancer of the testicle is not uncommon, I have seen my share of tragedies. Some patients handle their cruel fate extraordinarily well, while others come apart. Strong religious faith appears to help, but not always, since some patients turn against everything—friends, family, and faith. Several case histories are memorable.

A.C. was a twenty-eight-year-old senior medical student. While on a rotation in Boston, he noticed a hard lump in his right testicle. There was no pain, no urinary disturbance, not even a feeling of being unwell. He consulted the doctors at the Boston hospital, who all thought he needed immediate surgery. He elected to return home and came directly from the airport to see me. He was apologetic about disturbing me and, despite his apprehension, was calm and personable. He was going to make one fine physician. On examination, there was a stony, hard lump in the body of the testicle, and there could be no doubt that the medical student had cancer of the testicle.

I confessed my suspicion and we agreed to an immediate course of action, which involved hospitalization, the drawing of blood for markers, and an immediate operation.

The removal of the testicle was a simple fifteen-minute procedure. We looked for clues about the seriousness of the cancer at surgery. Did the tumor extend beyond the testicle? Was there a hemorrhage within the organ? We examined the testicle under the microscope.

In this case, we got back the best report possible—the tumor was a pure seminoma. In fact, seminoma is the most common form of this malignancy. It occurs in the widest age range, looks like fish flesh when cut open, and melts away under radiation. Its response to radiotherapy is so good that even when there is no suspicion of a spread, a course of radiotherapy is offered.

A.C. was older than most students, having worked as a research lab technician before becoming a med student. He was married, too, but had put off starting a family until he had graduated from medical school.

I had his sperm banked and gave him the course of radiotherapy. There has been no recurrence of the disease. After graduation, he interned on the West Coast. He became a father, with his frozen sperm, two years later. I'm curious to know if there is enough in the bank for another child. Theoretically, A.C.'s second child will be younger than the first in terms of the ovum, but just as old as the first as far as the sperm is concerned.

B.D., another memorable patient, was an angry young man by the time he came to see me. He had had a painful swelling in his left testicle for a month. The first consultant had told him that he had epididymitis. He had been treated with antibiotics and told to cut down on his sex life, which the doctor implied was the causative factor. The second consultant, seen just one week before he came to see me, had told B.D. that he had cancer. He was seeing me for a second opinion. A quick examination of the scrotal content left little doubt in my mind.

"I don't like the looks of this," I said. "I'm afraid I have to agree with Dr. X [the second consultant]."

"Damn it," he said, "I'm twenty-six and I'm going to die."

"There's no need to be so pessimistic," I said, trying to be reassuring.

"But I didn't tell you, Doc, they also found something in my chest X ray," the young man said.

I was furious with him. Why the hell hadn't he told me? Why was he wasting time getting opinions when he needed treatment? I was mad as hell, all right, but he sensed that a lot of my anger was directed not at him, but at the disease.

"I'm not stupid," he said. "Do you see any point in chopping off my ball when the disease is already in my lung?"

I was taken aback. It is true that removal of the primary site, when the disease has already spread, may not affect prognosis.

"We need to know what kind of tumor it is so that we can offer appropriate treatment."

"Why don't you assume the worst and get on with the chemotherapy? That's what you guys want me to agree to, isn't it?"

"You know, you have a perfectly valid argument. In fact, if this were any other tumor, I might completely agree with you. You are concerned that cutting you up may spread the disease, that the surgery and the anesthetic may weaken you, that the procedure may be more academic than therapeutic. But you are wrong! We need to know what kind of tumor you have. If you're lucky, it will be a seminoma and you will respond to radiotherapy. If it's a chorio or an embryonal, you're going to need cyclical chemotherapy."

"Will you look after me?" he asked.

"You saw Dr. X first—don't you think you should go back to him?"

"I don't like the way he reacted to my questions."

"You do have a way with questions," I said, and agreed to be his doctor.

The tumor turned out to be one of the nasty ones—an embryonal cell carcinoma that was already in his lungs. I consulted my oncologist friend (a doctor who specializes in cancer chemotherapy) and I visited while B.D. went through numerous courses of chemotherapy. He had the works: vinblastine, Actinomycin-D, bleomycin, cisplatin, cyclophosphamide, and Adriamycin. His hair fell out. He retched and vomited, lost weight, looked cadaverous. Then he got better, put on weight, and raised false hopes. He died less than two years after his first visit. I remember our last conversation.

"Thanks, Doc," he whispered, "and I'm not mad at you because you talked me into submitting to your scalpel." To this day I am upset that I did not have him fully convinced that we had to have a tissue diagnosis. There was a chance things might have turned out differently—B.D. was unlucky. The drugs used in cancer chemotherapy are all poisonous to the human body. It is simply that they are slightly more poisonous to cancer cells than they are to most normal cells. Normal cells of the type that replace themselves rapidly (such as white blood cells, cells from the intestinal lining, and cells from the roots of the hair) are vulnerable to anticancer drugs. Thus during chemotherapy there is an increased risk of infection due to the depletion of the white blood cells. There is nausea, vomiting, and bleeding from the intestinal tract due to the excess shedding of cells. And because the cells of the hair roots are damaged, there is loss of hair.

The oncologist treads a fine line between killing cancer cells and preserving normal cells. His therapeutic objectives are usually achieved by using a combination of drugs, in rotation. As experience increases, protocols for effective treatment are becoming more and more standardized.

R.M. was a thirty-four-year-old civil servant when I first met him. He had a charming and beautiful wife, a social worker by profession. They were an attractive couple, the kind you would expect to be surrounded by children. But they were childless. And not by choice.

He had been born with undescended testicles on both sides. At age five, both testicles were brought down, but there was a complication on the right side and the right testicle had been removed. Now, the repositioned and remaining left testicle harbored a suspicious lump. The odds were that the lump was malignant.

After blood markers were drawn, the left testicle was removed. The pathology report indicated a teratocarcinoma, apparently confined to the testicle.

A lymph-node dissection followed. This operation generally follows the finding of a tumor reported to be an embryonal cell carcinoma or a teratocarcinoma. The principle is that cancer spreads from the testicle into the draining lymph nodes before it seeds into other tissue, such as the lungs or liver. If we are able to remove the cancerous node or nodes, so the reasoning goes, we have a chance of arresting the disease before it seeds into other tissue. In reality, the disease has, with rare exceptions, already spread beyond the regional lymph nodes once it has invaded the nodes, and it may be that in most cases, the lymph-node dissection is an unnecessary trauma.

The lymph-node dissection is a major assault on the body. The body is cut down the center from the level of the lower margin of the breast bone to the level of the pubic bone. The abdomen is opened and the entire contents pushed aside so that the posterior lining can be cut through. This is where the major blood vessels, the aorta and vena cava, lie. Both vessels and their branches are stripped of adherent fat and fibrous tissue which are intermixed with the lymph nodes. The operation has its share of complications. For one thing, stripping the artery strips the sympathetic nerve fibrils, and this results in a backflow of the semen into the bladder upon ejaculation.

Patients who are not subjected to the staging lymph-node dissec-

107

tion are followed carefully and started on chemotherapy whenever there is a suggestion of a lump on ultrasound or on a CT scan, or if the blood markers are elevated. Elevated levels of alpha-fetoprotein are a sign that embryonal-cell-carcinoma cells or teratocarcinoma cells somewhere in the body are secreting the chemicals. Elevated levels of beta-HCG indicate the presence of live choriocarcinoma cells. Certain seminoma cells secrete this hormone as well, however, confusing the issue.

R.M. survived the lymph-node dissection and all his lymph nodes were free of disease. One year later, though, a three-centimeter lump overlying the lower aorta was detected on ultrasound and confirmed by CT scan. Surgical exploration uncovered a node missed at the time of lymph-node dissection. A course of chemotherapy was administered after the lump was removed. So far, four years later, R.M. remains free of detectable disease, but he lives with Damocles' sword over his head.

One might wonder if it is not more logical to defer lymph-node dissection in all cases and to proceed with chemotherapy at the first suggestion of nodal disease. Although chemotherapy may become the standard treatment, doctors who treat this disease in large numbers are not yet prepared to make this proposal. They point out, instead, that lymph-node dissection is free of major complications and appears to arrest progression of the cancer in acceptable numbers. They point out, in addition, that chemotherapy is not without hazards.

H.L. was a twenty-one-year-old engineering student when he first noticed that something was wrong. He started to develop breasts. Not the kind of fat that chubby boys acquire, but glandular, pubescent girl's breasts. His doctor referred him to an endocrinologist (a hormone specialist) who tested his blood and found the level of the beta human gonadotropin sky-high. He was sent to me with the presumptive diagnosis of a testicular tumor.

I examined H.L. thoroughly but could find nothing wrong with his testicles. I called the endocrinologist and told him that I had found nothing.

"Are you sure?" he asked. "There's not much else that can cause that kind of reading. His HCG was was beyond recording on the machine."

So we launched a head-to-toe examination, and finally, the diagnosis was made on ultrasound. A mass the size of a tennis ball was detected where the artery and vein of the right kidney are located. A CT scan confirmed the presence of the mass and, more importantly, detected no other mass.

At surgery, the lump dissected off the renal artery and vein very nicely, but it was attached to the vena cava. The vein, three centimeters in diameter, had to be clamped above and below the site of attachment. The "tennis ball" would not come off the vena cava without taking part of the vein wall with it. And no wonder. The tumor had extended through the wall of the vein and protruded inside the vena cava. If pieces of the tumor had not come off and seeded throughout the body, they were surely about to do so. When what remained of the vena cava was closed, the normal three centimeters were narrowed to pencil size. The student's recovery was remarkable. The HCG levels dropped dramatically. By the time the first course of chemotherapy had been completed, the markers were normal.

Six months later, a repeat ultrasound study of the testicles found a tiny spot in his right testicle. The right testicle was removed. The pathologist could find only a microscopic scar with no evidence of tumor cells, and we will never know if the removal was necessary or not. Undoubtedly, though, this was where the cancer had started. Now, three years later, the young man is alive and well.

I have described four cases from my practice. They were selected because each was memorable, but, in sum, they reflect the kind of optimism that now pervades the field. Three out of four patients are alive. Twenty years ago, after a diagnosis of choriocarcinoma, not one patient would have survived the year.

When there is talk about the "war against cancer," there is too much emphasis on failure—our failure to understand the cause, our failure to cure with surgery, or radiotherapy, or chemotherapy. We overlook the triumphs. Today we can expect to cure ninety percent of all cancers of the testicles. Progress in the treatment of cancer of the testicles, as well as in the control of leukemia, lymphoma, and Hodgkin's disease, to name a few, are truly miraculous by any standards. When our society becomes more curious about the working conditions of underfunded researchers, we shall see even greater progress. If a doctor is amply rewarded for restoring the health of one patient, how much more valuable is the work of scientists whose discoveries improve the health of the world?

Can I get a "truss" instead of having the hernia operation?

A truss is a padded belt on a metal frame. It supports the weak area in the lower abdominal wall through which the hernia protrudes. When it is fitted correctly and worn properly, it can control a relatively small hernia. On the other hand, I have seen men with a truss that is neither supporting the wall, nor containing the hernia. Some men manage to avoid hernia repair for years by using a truss, but they are only dealing with the symptom. There is no cure for a hernia other than surgical repair. Since younger people are less likely to have complicating health problems, it is wise not to delay the operation too long. If a patient wishes to avoid or to postpone the surgery at any cost, and if the hernia can readily be held in by a truss, there is no reason why it should not be tried.

Should I have my hernia repair with a local or a general anesthetic?
A local anesthetic avoids the lung complications associated with a general anesthetic, such as a pneumonia or a partially collapsed lung. On the other hand, if large amounts of the local anesthetic are necessary, excess amounts may be absorbed into the body, creating cardiac irregularities. The fluid can also distort the anatomy and interfere with the repair.

Is it possible that my hydrocele will get better on its own?
If the fluid is able to flow into the abdominal cavity, the hydrocele can disappear. This is known as a communicating hydrocele and is, unfortunately, uncommon.

Why does a varicocele cause distress in some men and not in others?
A slowly developing varicocele will not cause any symptoms. A rapidly developing one will, but the degree of distress varies from person to person.

110

We've just found out that our fifteen-year-old has an unde-scended testicle. What should we do?
Most experts advise removal and replacement of the testicle with a prosthesis. I might advise surgical correction rather than removal in cases in which the testicle was relatively low and could easily be returned to its proper position in the scrotum. It would be necessary to follow the surgery with careful ultrasound testing for potential testicular cancer.

Why don't you do a biopsy before you remove a testicle only suspected of containing a cancer?
On occasion, when the suspicion of cancer is not certain, the blood vessels going to and from the organ are first "soft-clamped" in the groin, the testicle pulled out of the scrotum and through the wound, and a biopsy specimen obtained for frozen section examination. A biopsy that doesn't interrupt the blood flow is never done because it might spread cancer cells into the bloodstream.

Is there any way to avoid going bald while undergoing chemo-therapy?
No, but it is certain that the hair will grow back.

Can a person die from chemotherapy for a testicular tumor?
Yes, but not likely. The threat to life is much, much greater from the cancer, and there is no doubt that chemotherapy cures the vast majority of patients with testicular cancers.

Can a person regain fertility after a course of chemotherapy?
It is possible, but cannot be predicted. Sperm banking, when pos-sible, is the best precaution.

Does a man lose his potency after chemotherapy?
It is possible, but not likely. The testosterone-producing cells of the testicle are not easily damaged. A temporary state of impotence can result from the weakened condition.

8 SEXUALLY TRANSMITTED DISEASES

A generation ago, an infectious disease acquired from sexual contact was called a venereal disease. Two of these diseases, syphilis and gonorrhea, became well known by the public. There was much less familiarity with the other so-called venereal diseases: chancroid, lymphogranuloma venereum, and granuloma inguinale, because they were considered tropical diseases and, therefore, less relevant to people of the Western world.

The old term "venereal disease" has been replaced by the term "sexually transmitted disease," or STD. STD includes a much wider collection of illnesses than did the old category. Included in the group are chlamydia, trichomonas, genital herpes, genital warts, and AIDS (acquired immune deficiency syndrome). There are other illnesses that may or may not be sexually transmitted, such as yeast infections, bacterial vaginitis, scabies, pubic lice, hepatitis B, and cancer of the cervix. This chapter attempts to clarify all available information on STD.

Today, men and women have little fear of the traditional venereal diseases because they know that modern medicine can almost always cure them. What people do fear, to the point of paranoia and hysteria, is genital herpes, because a cure is uncertain, and AIDS, because it can kill. There is less concern about the other sexually transmitted diseases, although they, too, have disturbing effects.

SYPHILIS Effective treatment for syphilis has only been available for the last fifty years, but the scourge of syphilis has been around for centuries. The English called it the

French disease; the French, I suspect, called it the English disease. Every country had it, and no country had a cure for it.

The causative microorganism cannot be seen under an ordinary microscope, but it can be identified, using a special microscope, by means of a technique called darkfield illumination. The effect is like looking into a darkroom in which the bacteria appear as dancing lights, unique in their large size and spiral shape. This microscopic identification is important because *Treponema pallidum*, the bacteria which cause syphilis, cannot be grown in the laboratory for purposes of identification.

The syphilis bacteria are transferred from an infected person to an uninfected person through sexual intercourse. In general, not much happens for three weeks after exposure, but the incubation period can be as little as ten or as long as sixty days. Then a sore, with distinct features, appears at the site where the bacteria have invaded their new host.

This sore, called a chancre, looks like a miniature crater with rough, hard edges. The surface of the crater is pink and oozes a watery discharge. There may be one or several of these sores, and there are painless enlarged lymph nodes nearby in the groin. These nodes are readily palpable to the examining fingers. This primary stage, with its sore or sores, lasts one to five weeks.

After the sore or sores have healed, there may be no obvious evidence of any disease for two to ten weeks. Then a widespread measles-like rash appears and lasts for days, only to disappear completely without treatment. This rash is called the secondary stage. Untreated patients may get attacks of the rash for up to two years.

The disease then enters what is called the latent phase. During the first two years of this period the patient is infectious, but after two years there is almost no chance of passing on the disease. During this latent period, which can last a lifetime, there may be no further evidence of the disease, or there may be signs of progressive disease in different parts of the body. There can be heart disease, mainly of the aorta; blood vessel disease, usually a blowout of an artery; damage to the spinal cord, at the place where sensations from the legs are carried to the brain; and brain damage that is commonly associated with dementia.

The diagnosis is made by looking for the bacteria in the watery discharge of the primary sore and, indirectly, by checking for the

113

antibodies in the blood, which appear about five weeks after the initial exposure. The blood test is known as the VDRL test.

The VDRL (Venereal Disease Research Laboratory) is the most common blood test, but it is not totally accurate. One out of four patients will test negative in the early stages of the disease. Some people will test positive not because they have syphilis, but because of malaria, leprosy, lupus, and even after a smallpox vaccination.

Syphilis is simply treated with penicillin, 2.4 million units once weekly for three weeks, intramuscularly. When the patient is allergic to penicillin, tetracycline or erythromycin at a dosage of one 500-milligram tablet four times a day for fifteen days is prescribed and is equally effective. If there are neurological complications, often intravenous antibiotics over an extended period of time are required. The effectiveness of the treatment is signaled by changes in the antibodies in the blood. It is not uncommon for antibodies to remain in the blood for three or four years after treatment, although the carrier is not contagious. It is best if the disease is diagnosed and treated in its primary stage, but progression can be halted when the disease is treated even in its secondary or tertiary stage.

GONORRHEA The bacteria which cause gonorrhea may be less damaging to the many different organs of the body than those of syphilis, but they have an insidious capacity to thrive and multiply in the moist, oxygen-deprived lining of the urethra of men and women. Laboratories that grow the *Neisseria gonorrhoeae* bacteria must duplicate these conditions. In the old days, labs grew the bacteria on a blood-and-gelatin surface in a culture jar that was depleted of its oxygen by having a lighted candle burn out inside it. If the environment is not moist and oxygen-deprived, the bacteria die. That explains why health care professionals often laugh when patients suggest that their infection was acquired from a toilet seat or from a swimming pool. More likely, since this bacteria can live in the genital tract of some men and women without causing symptoms, the cause is a silent carrier.

The incubation period for gonorrhea ranges from one day to fourteen days, but can be longer. As a rule, the shorter the incubation period, the more virulent the attack. Half the people infected will have a copious green and yellow discharge—from the urethra in men and from the vagina in women. Twenty-five percent will have a discharge more like that seen in other forms of urethritis, that is, more watery. Twenty-five percent will have no symptoms at all and become the silent carriers.

The diagnosis of gonorrhea is established microscopically by examining the gonorrhea bacteria within the white blood cells in the discharge. The bacteria is known as a Gram-negative diplococcus, which means that when a smear on a microscope slide is stained with Gram's stain, the bacteria appear red rather than blue, and they appear in pairs. The diagnosis is confirmed by growing bacteria in the laboratory from a swab taken from the urethra or vagina.

Most cases of gonorrhea respond to penicillin (4.8 million units into any muscle along with one gram of probenecid by mouth). Probenecid prolongs the action of penicillin by blocking its elimination from the kidney. Amoxicillin can be given by mouth three grams all at once, along with one gram of probenecid. Amoxicillin is a new form of penicillin, equally effective and preferred by people who abhor needles. Tetracycline (500 milligrams by mouth four times a day for two weeks) can be substituted when there is an allergy to penicillin and/or amoxicillin. A rare strain of the bacteria produces a chemical that inactivates penicillin; this strain has to be treated with another antibiotic called spectinomycin (two grams intramuscularly).

A swab from the urethra, one inch from the opening, should be cultured a week after treatment to ensure that the disease has been successfully eradicated. Gonorrhea can and should be cured in all instances.

Every new case of gonorrhea must be reported to the health authorities. The health officials trace all contacts. Only in this way can we eliminate the silent pool of carriers who are the greatest threat in spreading the disease. The judicious use of condoms can also help contain the spread of gonorrhea.

TROPICAL VENEREAL DISEASES Tropical venereal diseases are exceptionally rare in the Western world. The three cases I have seen in over twenty years of practice have been carried by visitors from tropical countries. For anyone unfortunate enough to acquire one of these illnesses, it is encouraging to remember that all are responsive to commonly used antibacterial agents.

Chancroid

This disease is caused by a bacteria called *Hemophilus ducreyi*. The incubation period of chancroid ranges from three to ten days. A low-grade fever and malaise may then occur, followed by an ulcer like that seen in syphilis except that the edges are soft, and the enlarged lymph nodes in the groin are painful and tender, unlike those seen in syphilis. The disease responds to sulfonamide (tri-methoprim-sulfamethoxozole double-strength tablet twice a day for ten days). Tetracycline or erythromycin can be substituted for the sulfonamide when there is intolerance or allergy to the sulfa.

Lymphogranuloma Venereum

This venereal disease is caused by a particular strain of the chlamydia bacteria. The incubation period ranges from three to fourteen days. The most characteristic feature of this disease is that the lymph nodes in the groin enlarge to such an extent that they mat together, invade and turn the overlying skin purple, and then break through to the outside. The disease is treated with sulfonamides, tetracycline, or erythromycin.

Granuloma Inguinale

This disease has features of the two previously described diseases —large matted nodes in the groin and soft-edged ulcers. It is caused by another family of bacteria, called *C. granulomatis*. The disease has an incubation period ranging from eight to eighty days, and it responds to the standard antibiotic treatment previously described.

CHLAMYDIA URETHRITIS

Chlamydia urethritis used to be difficult to diagnose because the standard laboratory technique for culturing bacteria is not effective in this case. We had to grow the bacteria in a lab inside live cells, as we did with viruses. Recently, commercial detection kits have become available. The test detects chlamydial protein by binding it to a prepared antibody that is linked to an enzyme. When the antibody is taken up, the enzyme changes color. Until this identification was made, clear urethral discharge not attributable to gonorrhea was called nonspecific urethritis, an inflammation of the urethra associated with discharge. Now, it is known that the chlamydia bacteria is responsible for most cases of nonspecific urethritis and, also, for most cases of epididymitis, which is a painful swelling of the epididymis. In women, chlamydia infection is a major cause of spontaneous abortion, tubal pregnancy, pelvic inflammatory disease, and infertility.

But fifty percent of all cases of chlamydial infections are totally free of any symptoms. In a study of eight hundred women who had come for their annual Pap smear at a government health center in Montreal, seven and a half percent had chlamydia without knowing it. The infection was seen twice as often in women who were under twenty-five years of age, and who had a red cervix or had inflammatory findings on their Pap test. Thus it might be prudent for men and women who are sexually promiscuous to have themselves tested for the chlamydial organism.

The fifty percent who develop symptoms do so after an incubation period of one to three weeks. These men and women experience a burning sensation while urinating and develop a discharge which is sticky and clear to creamy in color.

Treatment of chlamydial infection is simple enough, however. The disease responds to tetracycline, five hundred milligrams four times a day for ten to fourteen days. Other medications that can be used as well include erythromycin, second-generation tetracyclines such as Vibramycin or minocycline, and the sulfonamides such as the trimethoprim-sulfamethoxozole combination.

UREAPLASMA   Ureaplasma is an unusual and confusing bacteria. It has no cell wall, as do most bacteria, but it is sensitive to antibiotics, which is not the case with a virus. In recent years, microbiologists have developed a specific test for ureaplasma. The problem is, if you have it, do you treat it?

Seventy percent of people with ureaplasma have no problems. Some have symptoms which come and go over the years. Others have experienced miscarriage, infection of the tubes, and infection of the epididymis, and the only positive pathogen was ureaplasma.

Doctors researching the field treat ureaplasma only when three conditions pertain: when they can see signs of infection; when the patient reports symptoms; and when all the other tests for STDs are negative and only the ureaplasma test is positive.

Signs of infection in women are a red cervix and a puslike discharge from the cervix. Symptoms in women are: a transparent vaginal discharge (lots or a little), burning when urinating, and discomfort during sexual relations because the vaginal skin becomes delicate and fragile due to the discharge. In men there may be a clear discharge from the penis.

The treatment used today is tetracycline. Based on a culture after a course of treatment, seventy-five to eighty-five percent of the patients are cured. Oddly enough, however, patients often report the same symptoms despite this treatment. Tetracyclines are strong and often cause stomach upset. Lab data suggests that a new family of antibiotics, called quinolones, are a promising agent for ureaplasma. Although there are, as yet, no clinical studies on the use of quinolones for ureaplasma, studies on the use of quinolones for chlamydia, a similar bacteria, show a cure rate of seventy percent. Some people are free of symptoms after a period of time with no treatment at all. Sometimes the symptoms reoccur and sometimes they do not. Treatment of ureaplasma is considered a gray area of medicine.

TRICHOMONAS   *Trichomonas vaginalis* is a common cause of a frothy, itchy, malodorous vaginal discharge in women. The responsible organism looks like a teardrop-shaped miniature water insect, because it has a flat body and a tail that causes it to wiggle under the microscope. It can live in the male genital tract in the urethra or prostate, but is often asymptomatic in men. Trichomonas can ping-pong between the sexes and is thus considered sexual in transmission. I have difficulty accepting a sexual cause in all cases, however, since I have seen the problem in sexually abstinent women, and furthermore it is disproportionately female. No reasonable explanation for this sex distribution has been offered. Recently, it has been reported that these unicellular organisms can survive for up to one day in towels, clothes, chlorinated water, hot tubs, and weak soap solutions, as well as forty-five minutes on a toilet seat, thus raising the possibility of nonsexual transmission.

The diagnosis is made by seeing the protozoa, a unicellular organism of differing shapes and complex life cycles, under the microscope. Treatment consists of a drug called metronidazole (Flagyl), which is taken as a vaginal suppository or as a 250-milligram pill three times a day for ten to fifteen days by both partners. Flagyl is known to have caused cancer in rats, but whether it can promote cancer in humans is unknown. I feel that the drug presents a very slight risk, but I recommend it to a patient who has trichomonas since it is the only drug we know that combats trichomonas. The drug, however, is considered too dangerous for women to take during early pregnancy because of increased risk of a malformed baby.

VENEREAL WARTS The scientific name for a venereal wart is condyloma accuminata. As with all other warts, the cause is a virus which, as might be suspected, can easily be passed from one person to another by intimate sexual relations.

The wart looks like a tiny pink cauliflower and is easily recognized in men. It is much more difficult to see in women because the wart is similar in color to the vaginal wall and because the corrugations of the vagina camouflage the wart. In men, the warts can be located on the head of the penis, on the shaft of the penis, on the scrotum, around the anus, at the opening of the urethra, and even inside the urethra. In women, the warts can be near the clitoris, on the outer or inner lips, around the anus, at the opening of the vagina, even deep inside the vagina, and on the cervix. There can be tremendous variation in the size of the warts, ranging in size from a few millimeters to a few centimeters. If there has been mouth-to-genital contact, there can be warts inside the mouth in either sex.

Venereal warts can be treated in a number of ways. A chemical called podophyllin can be applied directly to the wart. Commonly, a twenty percent solution of the drug, mixed with tincture of benzoin to make it sticky, is dabbed on the wart and the centimeter of skin surrounding it and left on for a minute. It is then neutralized by an application of rubbing alcohol. The podophyllin treatment can be acutely painful when applied to delicate tissue such as the urinary opening or the head of the penis.

The warts can be burned off with an application of frozen nitrogen, by electrocautery, or with a laser. The frozen nitrogen method burns an area larger than necessary, and electrocautery requires some form of anesthetic. The laser treatment will eventually become

119

the treatment of choice as it is totally painless, but most hospitals are not yet equipped for it. Improperly applied laser treatment can cause horrendous complications, as in the case of a man who required skin grafting to cover the burned area and who remains impotent from damage to the nerve that runs in the midline on the top of the penis and which is responsible for all normal sensations from the penis.

When the warts are inside the male urethra, overly aggressive treatment such as that done with electrocautery can cause a stricture of the passage. Weekly instillations of the anticancer drugs, 5-fluorouracil or thiotepa, instead, have successfully eradicated the warts after about five treatments. When the wart is on the cervix of women, it is often wise to perform a biopsy as venereal warts have been linked to the development of cervical cancer.

Even when there is no longer any visible evidence of venereal warts, they can reoccur without reexposure. And when long neglected, giant warts measured in inches may cover the genitalia. These are associated with cancer formation at the site.

I remember using electrocautery and general anesthetic to burn off innumerable venereal warts around the genitalia and anus of one patient, and then, remembering that there was another one inside the mouth, I moved to the head of the table and applied the instrument to the wart inside the mouth. The nurse, watching me, was alarmed. "You just used that instrument on the guy's bum!" she exclaimed. "I know," I replied, "but it's all right, electrocautery is self-sterilizing." She gave me a look of utter disgust. I don't know if it was my technique that did it or the nature of this particular health problem.

I advise my patients to check themselves for warts for as long as one year after successful eradication. As the incubation period for condyloma can be as long as six months, I consider it cured only after one whole year free from new warts.

HERPES   Genital herpes is the third most common sexually transmitted disease today. Gonorrhea is still number one and chlamydia is number two.

The causative organism is a herpes simplex virus which exists in two forms, called type 1 and type 2, with only a minor chemical difference between them. The type 1 virus is associated ninety percent of the time with blisters around the mouth and ten percent of the time with blisters on the genitals. The type 2 virus is associated ninety percent of the time with blisters on the genitals, and ten percent of the time with blisters on the mouth.

The herpes virus can be transferred from an infected person onto the skin or genital lining of an uninfected person by intercourse or sexual play. There is a two- to ten-day incubation period. During this time, there may be pain and a pins-and-needles feeling at the site of the viral transfer. Then, flulike symptoms develop—fever, headaches, malaise, muscle aches, and swollen lymph nodes. Later, at the site of transfer, tiny blisters appear on a reddened base. In women, the blisters occur on the vulva, vagina, and cervix; in men, the common sites are the head of the penis, foreskin, and shaft of the penis. After a week or two, the blisters burst and become tiny, painful erosions or ulcers. A dry crust forms over the ulcers about twenty days later. Between the time the blisters break and the time they crust over, the virus is contagious and can be transmitted to others.

It takes about three weeks for herpes ulcers to heal. After this time, the painful, enlarged lymph nodes, which have developed in the groin, also subside and the attack is over.

But even when there is no further evidence of an attack, the virus remains in the body, inside the nerve cells. Attacks recur in eighty percent of patients, but they are usually milder than the first episode.

The diagnosis is made by simple inspection. If there is any doubt, the diagnosis can be double-checked by scraping material from the base of the blister, staining it, and examining it under a microscope. The scraping contains giant cells with many nuclei. These giant cells are also seen in chicken-pox scrapings and in shingles, but there is little confusion with these illnesses when the overall picture is considered. The diagnosis can also be confirmed by viral tissue culture.

There is no curative treatment for genital herpes. A drug called acyclovir was introduced in 1985. It does not kill the virus, but does slow its rate of reproduction. Acyclovir cream applied to the blisters decreases pain and shortens the duration of the attack. It is considered effective for the first attack, but of questionable value for subsequent attacks. Acyclovir pills have also hit the market. Two-hundred-milligram tablets taken every four hours for ten days lessen the severity of the attack and speed up healing. Frequent recurrent attacks may also be lessened by taking the pills three times a day for as long as six months. In the short time acyclovir has been available, there has been no report of any dangerous side effects, but the medication is expensive.

A young lady once asked me if I approved or disapproved of her starting a relationship with a man who had a history of genital herpes. I told her that the safest procedure would be to use a condom at all times. If she did not use a condom when her lover had blisters, she was taking an enormous risk. When he was blister-free, the risk was small but still existed. I figured, though, that a caring relationship transcends an illness like herpes, which is never fatal.

AIDS Statistics and information on AIDS (acquired immune deficiency syndrome) are continually changing, and it is difficult to have perspective in the middle of an epidemic. At this time, in early 1988, over one hundred countries are affected by the disease and *several million people* have contracted the virus. According to the World Health Organization, more than 120,000 cases of AIDS have been reported since the discovery of the virus in 1981, and *five to ten million people are carriers of the virus*. In the United States, the cities most affected are New York and San Francisco. By the most conservative estimates of the New York City Health Commissioner, *five hundred thousand* people in the metropolitan New York area carry the antibodies to AIDS. By the end of 1987, over thirty thousand Americans had developed AIDS. It has already become the first cause of death for women between twenty and twenty-five and men between twenty-five and forty in New York City. One and a half million Americans and countless millions of Africans now carry antibodies to the AIDS virus.

The control of this epidemic will depend on the development of a vaccine or a drastic change in sexual habits. The U.S. Surgeon General estimated that it would take another thirty years to develop an effective vaccine. This is because the AIDS virus mutates and, like the flu virus, each new strain requires a separate vaccine. Since it took twenty years to develop a vaccine against hepatitis B, it is expected that a vaccine for this even more complicated virus will take longer.

It is difficult to know whether the general population is frightened enough of the AIDS epidemic to modify its sexual behavior, but

122

partner screening and the use of the condom appear imperative in controlling the epidemic.

Recovering the virus from infected tissue and growing it in tissue culture may seem the most logical way to study this disease. Theoretically, this is possible, but it is not often done since the culture technique is difficult, expensive, and generally unavailable. But the spin-off from the massive research effort to discover a cure for AIDS will likely advance our understanding of other disease processes such as cancer and transplantation rejection. A breakthrough in cancer control might well become the serendipitous bonus of this modern-day scourge.

The first case of AIDS in America was reported in 1981. Since then, AIDS has become the most serious epidemic of the last fifty years.

The causative virus has now been isolated and characterized. This virus, originally designated as HTLV-111 (human T-lymphotropic virus-111) in the United States and LAV (lymphadenopathy-associated virus) in France, is now internationally known as HIV (human immunodeficiency virus).

Right now there is no simple test that tells whether or not a person has AIDS. What is usually tested, instead, is whether or not a person has been exposed to the AIDS virus and has developed antibodies. Ninety-five percent of the people who have had a sexual or blood contact with the AIDS virus produce detectable levels of the antibody. Five percent do not produce antibodies, even though they have the AIDS virus. The ELISA test (enzyme-linked immunosorbent assay) is the blood test used to determine the presence of antibodies. When antibodies are present, a reaction occurs which changes the color of the enzyme linked to them.

Historically, the people with the most risk of AIDS were homosexuals, intravenous drug users who shared needles, Haitians, hemophiliacs, and any blood product recipients. This has changed to some extent in that blood transfusions are now safer. All donations at blood donor clinics are screened for AIDS antibodies with the ELISA test, and blood that tests positive is obviously not used. Unfortunately, the test does not identify exposed donors who have not yet developed antibodies, nor does it screen out the five percent who have the virus without antibodies. Nevertheless, since the Red Cross began testing donors, there have been virtually no cases of transmission due to transfusion.

The AIDS virus is transmitted through blood, semen, and cervical-vaginal secretions. It has been found in urine, breast milk, tears, and saliva, but there has not yet been a documented case of transmission from these sources. The virus has been transmitted perinatally from infected mother to child during or shortly after birth. It used to be thought that the AIDS virus was transmitted only through anal intercourse. Now, it is known to be transmitted through vaginal intercourse as well. No case of transmission through oral intercourse has yet been reported. Researchers have shown, however, that the AIDS virus behaves like the hepatitis B virus. And since hepatitis B has been transmitted by oral sex alone, from men to men, it is presumed that the AIDS virus can be transmitted by oral sex.

The AIDS virus is known to have been transmitted in a single encounter and is thought to be an easily transmitted virus. The odds of infection from a single encounter are not known.

Condoms are suggested as a barrier to transmission. The *Journal of the American Medical Association* published a laboratory study showing that the AIDS virus cannot pass through either a synthetic or natural-skin condom. A University of Miami clinical study also showed the protective value of condoms. When condoms were used, only one out of ten of the partners of AIDS patients developed antibodies. This is in striking contrast to the twelve out of fourteen partners who developed antibodies when condoms were not used. These condom studies suggest that continued sexual contact without preventative measures will result in AIDS transmission, and that sexual contact with barrier contraceptives is, short of abstinence, the safest means of protection known.

There have been reports in the popular magazines that a certain spermacide inactivates the AIDS virus, but there are no scientific studies to support this claim. In laboratory studies, the AIDS virus has been killed by detergents, soaps, alcohol, and sterilization. The most effective disinfectant in the studies is a 0.5 percent solution of hypochlorite, the chemical in laundry bleach.

Perhaps one of the most frightening aspects of AIDS has to do with possible silent transmission. A person can be incubating the virus, not have sufficient antibodies to test positive, and still transmit the disease.

As of December 1986, the total caseload of heterosexual trans-mission in the United States since 1981 was 1,079. In Canada it was 18. For the U.S.A. this represents four percent of the total number of cases; for Canada it represents two to three percent. In 1987 seven percent of new cases were due to heterosexual transmission. On the other hand, over ninety-five percent of all cases are homosexual or involve those who share needles.

On the positive side, scientists who have studied families living with AIDS patients have shown that, apart from actual intimate sexual contact, transmission does not occur. In the families studied, the virus has not been transmitted to children by hugging, kissing, or by sharing kitchen and bathroom facilities.

Progress of the Disease
People who have had contact with the AIDS virus will develop an-tibodies, or seroconvert, one week to six months later. This means that after a suspected contact, a person can check to see if he or she is infected by having the ELISA antibody test. If the test is positive, the person has been exposed; if negative, the person is probably not infected.

If a person tests positive on the ELISA test, it is repeated, and is reconfirmed in another test called the western blot. This test looks for a different protein in the AIDS virus. Even if both tests are positive, it does not necessarily mean the person will get AIDS: the tests do not confirm that the person is infectious or infected. They indicate that at one time or another, the person has been exposed to the AIDS virus. The only hard data we have on the percentage of people with antibodies who actually get AIDS is based on a three-year study of homosexual men in New York City. And 34.2 percent of these seropositive men developed AIDS. AIDS experts feel that many more of these subjects would have developed AIDS if the study had continued over a longer period of time. The current estimate is that thirty to seventy percent of those who are seropositive will develop AIDS. People are counseled on the presumption that testing positive for antibodies means they may transmit the disease.

A person may have the AIDS virus for many years without feeling

125

sick. Recent analysis of data collected in San Francisco since 1978 suggests that the risk of developing AIDS increases yearly after infection with the virus. Four percent of people who became infected with the AIDS virus developed the disease within three years; after five years the figure rose to fourteen percent, and after seven years to thirty-six percent. There is considerable speculation beyond the seven-year period, but no hard data.

When the AIDS symptoms appear, they may do so in a variety of ways.

Most often, the seropositive patient will develop what is called the AIDS-Related Complex (ARC) before developing full-blown AIDS. ARC is defined by a collection of symptoms and lab findings. The symptoms are a three-month history of any two of the following:

1. Fever in excess of 100.4 degrees Fahrenheit
2. Night sweats
3. Ten-pound weight loss (or ten percent reduction of body weight)
4. Diarrhea
5. Fatigue
6. Enlarged lymph nodes in more than two areas other than the groin

The lab findings can include:

1. Decreased red blood cells, decreased white blood cell count, decreased platelets (tiny blood cell products necessary for normal clotting)
2. Increased immune responses, such as gamma globulin, which is the protein base for all antibodies that fight disease
3. Failure to respond to the tuberculosis skin test and other skin tests

Often, the clinical manifestations are yeast infections, unexplained mouth infections, and/or shingles, which show up as painful, pigmented blisters on the body at the site of the nerve endings.

Some people who develop this complex may die from it. Others will go on to develop full-blown AIDS, which is always fatal.

Some patients get AIDS without any preliminary stages. They get a specific form of pneumonia (*Pneumocystis carinii*), or a specific form of cancer (Kaposi's sarcoma). This is because the HIV virus attacks a particular family of blood cells, called T-helper lymphocytes, which are indispensable in producing certain immune responses. If all the T-helper lymphocytes are destroyed, the body

126

cannot resist certain serious lung infections or fight against the cancerous process. The pneumonia in AIDS is like any other pneumonia except that it may prove more difficult to manage. The cancer in AIDS also behaves no differently.

A small percentage of seropositive patients get neurological symptoms when they get AIDS. In fact, some patients manifest only neurological symptoms—a progressive loss of cerebral function accompanied by motor and behavioral disturbances. In a study of patients with only neurological symptoms, half developed full-blown AIDS and half died without exhibiting any other signs of AIDS.

There are a number of other diseases which may be considered sexually transmitted because of the manner in which they are spread.

HEPATITIS Hepatitis B, for example, does not affect the sexual organs, but it spreads much like AIDS, and the resulting severe destruction of the liver can be fatal. Hepatitis B can certainly be acquired nonsexually by a contaminated needle or from blood, but the virus can also be transmitted sexually. Hepatitis B vaccine is available and should be taken by the sexual partners of people who have, or are carriers of, the virus. The vaccine is made from the plasma of patients with the hepatitis B virus. These patients are often gay, so the public is fearful that they may pick up the AIDS virus when they get the vaccine. In fact, this is not possible, but the concern is only one of many misconceptions about hepatitis B.

Long ago, doctors recognized only two kinds of viral hepatitis. One was called infectious hepatitis, which is now called hepatitis A, and the other was called serum hepatitis, which is now called hepatitis B. Today there are two more viral agents identified, one called non-A/non-B, and another called hepatitis D virus, which is an incomplete virus that causes disease only when the hepatitis B virus is also present.

Hepatitis A
The hepatitis A virus is acquired by eating or drinking food, water, milk, or shellfish contaminated by the virus. (The virus inside the shellfish may not be destroyed by cooking when the shell is intact.) There is an incubation period of four weeks, after which low-grade

fever, tiredness, loss of appetite, nausea, vomiting, headaches, and muscle aches appear. Within a week, the urine turns dark, the stool turns light, pain and discomfort develop in the upper abdomen where the liver is located, and the skin and the whites of the eyes turn yellow. After several weeks, most patients slowly recover and develop a lifetime immunity to further attacks.

Hepatitis B
Five percent of the Earth's population, or two hundred million people, are chronically infected with the hepatitis B virus. The virus has been found in the body secretions of these people—saliva, tears, sweat, semen, vaginal secretions, breast milk, urine, and feces. Most transmissions, however, are from contaminated needles, sexual intimacy, or are carried into the newborn through a contaminated birth canal.

Once the virus is acquired, the incubation period can vary from one to three months, and rarely up to six months. The incubation period is shorter when the virus is inoculated into a cut or a needle prick, and longer when the transmission is sexual or oral.

Hepatitis B infection can then take an acute or a chronic course. In the acute course, the clinical disease is like that of hepatitis A, and recovery occurs after two to three months. Five to ten percent of patients with the acute course will remain chronically infected with the virus. In the chronic course, the beginnings of the disease are blurred, and the malaise persists for a long time. Eventually, the liver may shrivel up, a condition called cirrhosis, or it may develop a cancer.

Hepatitis B can be prevented by a newly developed vaccine. The vaccine was developed from the plasma of hepatitis B carriers, who have a noninfectious viral-coat protein in their plasma. The plasma is boiled, chemically treated to remove other proteins, and mixed with formalin. These processes eliminate any possibility of contamination with the live AIDS virus, but retain the potential to function as the hepatitis B vaccine.

Protection from hepatitis B is due to the vaccinated person's ability to produce protective antibodies. A person in a debilitated state may not be able to produce the antibodies. Also, when there is an accidental exposure to the hepatitis B virus, such as an accident in the operating room, or a sexual exposure, and there may not be sufficient time to produce the antibody response, hyperimmune serum or serum from patients who have already produced the antibodies are used. Such a treatment can abort an attack.

SCABIES AND LICE   Scabies, known for its tremendous itchiness, is caused by a tiny "insect" that burrows just under the skin. Scabies can be spread from one person to another by sexual relations. Lindane lotion or cream popularly known as Kwell applied for ten to twelve hours is usually curative.

Pubic lice, also known for its itchiness, is caused by a mite that survives on pubic hair. Close contact can spread the lice from one person to another. Lindane can be used again, but skin application of a drug called piperonyl butoxide may be less irritating and equally effective.

YEAST INFECTION AND CANCER OF THE CERVIX   Yeast infection of the vulva and vagina is not uncommon in women. This can occur without sexual contact: in women taking an oral antibiotic, in diabetics, in women on the pill, and in women who do not routinely use cotton underwear. There is often an intense vaginal itch and a discharge that is thick, white, and cheesy. This de novo yeast infection can be passed on to the male partner, whose only symptom may be an increased redness in the head and shaft of the penis. An antifungal cream such as miconazole (Monistat 7), clotrimazole (Lotrimin or Mycelex), or nystatin (Mycostatin or Nilstat) is curative.

Another common cause of vaginal discharge in women is infection caused by the *Gardnerella vaginalis* bacteria. A telltale fishy odor after intercourse is a sign of this infection. It is not certain whether this infection can be transmitted to men.

Finally, a case can be made to suggest that carcinoma of the cervix may be sexual in origin. For example, it has been determined that not one case of cancer of the cervix appeared in ten thousand nuns who were sexually abstinent. There is, on the other hand, statistical evidence that the cancer occurs more frequently in women who have had multiple sex partners. However, a causative factor, presumably associated with the penis, has not been identified.

There are specialized STD clinics that provide a battery of tests. If you think you have a disease, it is wise to find such a clinic. With

129

blood tests that measure antibodies and genital swabs that collect organisms for culture, it is possible to know if you have gonorrhea, syphilis, chlamydia, hepatitis B, ureaplasma, or AIDS. It is not uncommon for STD tests to come back negative and for symptoms to persist. Sometimes this is a misdiagnosis, but in other cases the symptoms are a result of sexual guilt, heightened sensitivity, or other psychological distress. In most cases the tests tell you what you have.

In general, having fewer partners reduces the chances of STD. Being prepared and careful is also helpful (carry a condom). There are those who prefer to take their chances and tend to disease later, but AIDS puts a new meaning on this insouciance. One thing seems certain—the undeniable urge of people to relate sexually is stronger than the fear of disease.

QUESTIONS AND ANSWERS

Can I get herpes from a person with no obvious sores?
The risk of transmission is certainly reduced when there are no visible signs, but not totally eliminated. One to fifteen percent of people with type 2 herpes will transmit the virus without themselves having any visible signs. You can, therefore, be unknowingly infected by your sexual partners.

What is the difference between type 1 and type 2 herpes virus?
There is a very slight protein difference, detectable in refined laboratory tests. The striking difference is seen in the health problems which result: type 1 virus usually causes fever blisters of the lips; type 2 virus causes genital ulcers.

Will tetracycline cure me of chlamydia?
Yes. It works now, but it may not tomorrow. For example, it used to be that every case of gonorrhea was cured by penicillin. Now there are penicillin-resistant strains of gonorrhea, especially in Southeast Asia.

Should I take tetracycline instead of penicillin for gonorrhea?
Treatment with tetracycline would likely eliminate chlamydia infection which might have been acquired at the same time. But there are gonorrhea infections that resist both penicillin and tetracycline.

130

Could I have gotten venereal warts from something other than sexual contact?

Not likely. Stated another way, it has been shown that sixy percent of the partners of patients with condyloma develop a venereal wart within a three-month period. The incubation period for this virus ranges from one to six months.

I guess I don't have to worry about getting syphilis since it's been eradicated from the face of the earth?

This is simply not so. In certain areas of the world, such as Western Europe and North America, more new cases of syphilis are being diagnosed now than a generation ago.

Can I avoid STDs by scrubbing with soap and water after sexual relations?

No! The simplest and most reliable protection would be the use of a condom.

Haven't French scientists developed an effective treatment for AIDS, and isn't there a new drug that is supposed to be effective?

The French scientists' preliminary results suggested that the immunosuppressive drug Cyclosporin A might help patients with AIDS. Subsequent follow-up of the patients has discounted the early results.

A new drug, called AZT, is currently being tried. It appears to help prolong life but is far from being curative.

Can I sue somebody for knowingly transmitting an STD?

There are several cases of this nature before the courts. The decisions of the lower courts will, undoubtedly, be appealed and the final outcome will take years. I suspect that people who knowingly transmit STDs will be prosecuted. But asymptomatic carriers can be the source of disease and the question of their responsibility is a complicated one. Carriers of gonorrhea, herpes, and chlamydia can be asymptomatic. And these are the three most common STDs.

Is AIDS more contagious than hepatitis B?

The hepatitis B virus is much more contagious, but AIDS is deadly.

9 SEX AND SEX CHANGES

Human sexuality is the stuff of poems, songs, fantasy, and much befuddlement. I can't pretend to be an expert on the delicate or delicious aspects of sexuality, but I can review what we know about human sexual development. For example, how is the process of puberty experienced differently by boys and girls? Is an intact hymen a foolproof test of virginity? What are the pros and cons concerning replacement hormones for women who have had their menopause? Is there a male menopause? What's a transsexual and what's the lowdown on the much publicized sex-change operation?

A good place to start a discussion about the stages of human sexual growth is by describing the basic element of human sexuality—the chromosome.

CHROMOSOMES Chromosomes are the genetic blueprint of human beings. They define each person's sex and biological potential. Half come from the father and half from the mother. The human species has twenty-three pairs of chromosomes, including one pair of sex chromosomes which determine gender. The father may contribute either an X or a Y chromosome; the mother always contributes an X chromosome. When an X chromosome comes from the father and combines with an X chromosome from the mother, it creates an XX sex chromosome pattern in the infant and the baby is a genetic female. When the father contributes a Y chromosome, the resulting XY pattern produces a genetic male. The father's chromosome, therefore, determines the genetic sex of the child.

The Y chromosome causes the inner part of the primitive sex organ to become the testicle. This early testicle produces testosterone, which in turn stimulates the appropriate primitive tissue to become the various male sex organs. In rare cases, when the male hormone is not available, even though there is an XY chromosome pattern, the baby will not develop male sex organs and will have the outward appearance of a girl. When the male hormone level is elevated, even a female baby will show more male features, such as an enlarged clitoris. When there are two X chromosomes, the outer part of the primitive gonad becomes the ovary and the baby develops both the internal and external sex organs of a girl.

Sometimes there is a problem with the inherited pattern of the sex chromosomes, as, for example, in Klinefelter's syndrome and Turner's syndrome. In Klinefelter's syndrome, the infant inherits an extra chromosome, ending up with an XXY pattern. This irregularity produces lanky arms, excess breast development, a penis with small testicles, and no sperm. In Turner's syndrome, another irregularity, the infant is missing a sex chromosome, ending up with an XO pattern. This person will look like a girl but will often be very short, with a webbed neck, no breasts, and nonfunctional ovaries.

Other bizarre patterns of chromosomal inheritance associated with infertility and frequent mental retardation do exist but these are rare. Most of us are born with straightforward XX or XY sex chromosomes. We are boys or girls. We may be infinitely various, but we will have a common evolutionary development—from child to adolescent, to adult, and perhaps to parenthood. And our first sex change will be that of puberty.

PUBERTY   The process of puberty is different for boys and girls, but in each case there are predictable physical changes.

The following are the changes normally seen in girls: There is a growth spurt at age twelve. Breast development may start as early as age eight or as late as age thirteen, and even later on occasion. Pubic hair appears, usually before menstruation, which, on the average, begins at age thirteen. All changes evolve gradually. The breast, for example, starts to bud. Then the pigmented area surrounding the nipple enlarges. Next the entire breast increases in size, the nipple and pigmented areas bulge, and finally the breast assumes its fully rounded adult appearance. Pubic hair changes from straight, sparse, and lightly pigmented to curly, coarser, pigmented hair in the shape of an inverted triangle. Menstruation is irregular at first and may not always be associated with ovulation.

A boy's growth spurt usually occurs around age fourteen. However, in boys the changes of puberty occur over a wider range than they do in girls. Boys experience a voice change, a deepening due to the thickening of the vocal cords. Their facial hair begins to grow. Muscle development increases; the scrotum, testicles, and penis gradually enlarge; and pubic hair appears, becomes thicker, and looks like a triangle pointing to the belly button. Also, fifty percent of all boys experience a breast enlargement which recedes within two years. All changes occur gradually over a two- to three-year period. The first ejaculation at about age fourteen is usually from masturbation or from nocturnal emission.

VIRGINITY AND SEX The loss of virginity and the beginning of an active sex life may be considered the next sex change. In boys there are no physical changes associated with the loss of virginity. In girls the hymen may be torn. Some people and certain societies place great emphasis on this change. In fact, the hymen is a rim of very ordinary tissue. I have been asked a number of times to reconstitute a torn hymen to simulate virginity. Although I have never carried out the procedure, gynecologists who do tell me that "virginity" is restored by stitching together the torn remnants of the hymen. To prevent unyielding scar tissue, the operation must be timed so that the hymen will be torn again a few days later.

MENOPAUSE Excluding childbirth, the menopause is the next major sexual change in women, and although it is a very important stage of a woman's life, most men know almost nothing about it.

Menopause is signaled by the cessation of menstruation. This occurs at about age fifty, but there is a wide age variation. As a rule, it is true that the earlier a woman begins to menstruate, the later she will finish.

Some women have no noticeable symptoms associated with menopause, yet others report symptoms such as diminished vaginal lubrication, irritation with urination, increased irritability, and depression. Two out of three women get hot flashes, which they describe as a sudden feeling of heat or redness in the face and upper body that lasts for several minutes. The hot flashes may recur from one to five years.

Most of the undesirable symptoms of menopause are attributable to a lack of estrogen, a hormone normally produced by the ovary. We do not know why the ovary produces less or no estrogen in middle age, but it does. Women who have a difficult menopause need their partner's understanding and support. Menopause is not a made-up or psychological disturbance. It is physiologically based.

Menopausal symptoms and disorders can all be lessened by the administration of estrogen. Skin changes, such as wrinkling and thinning, can be slowed down. Bone weakening, or osteoporosis, can be diminished, especially when combined with an adequate dietary intake of calcium. Vaginal and bladder infections also become less frequent.

But estrogen replacement therapy increases the risk of cancer of the uterine lining. The normal incidence is one in a thousand per year. When estrogen is administered, the risk is increased four times.

You might advise your partner that today gynecologists use a combination of estrogen and progesterone. This mixture most closely resembles normal female physiology and thus does not have the risks of estrogen alone. A number of studies have now confirmed that cancer of the uterine lining does not occur with any increased frequency in women treated with both hormones. But with the estrogen-progesterone combination, a woman still has her menstrual bleeding and this consequence may deter some women. If your partner has disagreeable menopausal symptoms and if she has had a hysterectomy, I would suggest estrogen replacement. If your partner wants treatment and still has her uterus, I would suggest a combination of estrogen and progesterone. Some women will want treatment and others will not. In either case, there is no diminishing of sexual desire because of menopause, and logistical problems, such

135

as lubrication, should they occur, can be treated. By all means continue sexual activity.

THE MALE MENOPAUSE The male menopause, or climacteric, supposedly occurring between forty-five and sixty-five, is, perhaps, more an intriguing concept than a scientific fact. It is defined in terms of a collection of symptoms: listlessness, poor appetite, weight loss, impaired ability to concentrate, weakness, irritability, depressed libido, and depressed erections. There is nothing very specific about these symptoms. Any man complaining of any or all of these symptoms could just as easily have anemia, depression, or an undiagnosed malignancy.

If there were a male counterpart to the female menopause, we should be able to demonstrate rather sudden lowered levels of circulating testosterone and a corresponding elevation in the pituitary gonadotropins at a particular period in life. The pattern that has been noted, instead, is a slow, gradual lowering of the testosterone level and an uneven loss of testicular tissue. Elderly men, even in their eighties and nineties, still have some testicular function and that explains why they can become fathers. Charlie Chaplin may be the most famous over-seventy-year-old father, but he is by no means the only one.

Male menopause is an intriguing concept, but not a likely reality. It is, perhaps, more to the point to look at stress and pressure as causes of unpleasant mid-life symptoms rather than to believe in this ethereal concept.

THE NORMAL SEX LIFE It is presumptuous to suggest what a "normal" sex life might be. Just as with exercise, diet, or fashion, what is right for one individual may be too much, or too little, for another. Nevertheless, there are surveys on the frequency of ejaculation and sexual intercourse within the life cycle and statements regarding the national "averages" can be made.

There is little doubt that, on the average, men in their early twenties have more ejaculations and sexual intercourse than at any other time of their lives. Women, generally, experience their strongest sex drive and most frequent orgasms in their late thirties. For men, the average frequency of ejaculation or intercourse per week during the twenties is four to five times; two to four times a week during the thirties; once or twice a week during the forties; none to once a week during the fifties. From the sixties on, frequency is most often expressed per month, and once or twice is the usual frequency quoted. In one survey, two thirds of men in their sixties were sexually active, as were one third of men in their seventies. Of course, sexual activity in these studies is defined only as ejaculation or intercourse, and many older people (to say nothing of homosexual women) consider this too narrow a definition of sexuality.

There is no doubt that men over the age of sixty take longer to achieve an erection, require more direct penile stimulation, have decreased firmness, and may experience less intensity with ejaculation. Also, after ejaculation, a longer time is necessary to reacquire an erection. But orgasms can be felt, even without ejaculation, and orgasms that are less intense may be totally sexually fulfilling. There is no question that with age the frequency of intercourse wanes, but not necessarily the sexual pleasure.

At any rate, I don't pay much attention to the "normal" figures. Often, when I provide them to patients, they happily conclude that their sexuality is livelier than the reported average. And my advice to an older man who wants to know why he isn't performing as frequently as his boastful neighbor is borrowed from a cartoon I once saw: "Well, no reason why you can't say the same thing."

SEXUAL IDENTITY   Admittedly, sexuality is a complex subject, and giving medical advice becomes more complicated when the disorder is psychological rather than physical. In these androgynous times, external appearances are often not enough to distinguish gender. Neither, even, are chromosomes if a person does not feel comfortable with his or her given sex. But science, undaunted, has developed a quantifiable way to assess gender.

Whether a person is male or female is medically defined in five ways:

1. In terms of whether the person has male or female chromosomes
2. In terms of whether the person has male or female internal sex organs (testicles, prostate, and seminal vesicles in men; ovaries, Fallopian tubes, uterus, cervix, and vagina in women)
3. In terms of the external sex organs (penis and scrotum in men; labia majora, labia minora, clitoris, and breasts in women)

4. In terms of the psyche
5. In terms of how the infant was raised—whether as a boy, or as a girl

Studies show that of these five criteria, the most important, psychologically, is how the infant was raised. Thus if a boy was accidentally, or deliberately, brought up as a girl, despite having external and internal male characteristics, he may feel himself to be a girl. In some cases, a person's sense of identity will best be served by altering his or her external appearance and becoming the opposite sex. In many other cultures and in ancient civilizations, sex change was simply accomplished by donning the attire and taking on the demeanor of the other sex. Since the 1950s, doctors have become involved in sex-change manipulation and now sex-change surgery is modern society's way of dealing with transsexuals.

THE SEX-CHANGE OPERATION

Male-to-Female

A male transsexual is one who feels he was born with the wrong sex. He is different from a male transvestite, who dresses in clothing of the opposite sex for sexual arousal, or a male homosexual, who prefers sexual relations with another male. The true transsexual wishes to alter himself physically, to actually be what he deeply feels is his true sexual identity. This means he must have a sex-change operation. Often a psychiatric assessment as to whether or not the applicant is a true transsexual is required before an operation is allowed. And on rare occasions, even the psychiatrist is fooled. There is a bond among the transsexual population and they may well discuss their pre-op interviews—what was asked and what the response should be.

Once a person is categorized as a true transsexual, treatment begins. First, estrogen, the female hormone, is taken by mouth. Electrolysis removes unwanted hair, and sometimes breasts are augmented by plastic surgery. This process of outward feminization can take up to two years. An operation to alter the external genitalia is then carried out.

A number of surgical techniques have been devised to create outer lips and a vagina. One procedure takes a short segment of large bowel and makes it into a vagina. Another uses a piece of skin taken from another part of the body and wraps it around a tubing to make a vagina. Possibly the most ingenious technique utilizes the skin of the penis to form the vagina, a procedure that seems to me to make the most sense.

After the patient is asleep, the legs are placed in stirrups and the body positioned as if for a prostate operation or for delivery of a baby. A catheter is inserted in the tip of the penis, through the urethra, and into the bladder. A cut is made around the circumference of the penis near the head. The skin covering the shaft of the penis is pushed down toward the body. The inside tissue, now bare, is removed carefully without damaging the urethra. The external skin of the penis is then pulled up and pushed back in on itself to make a vagina. This inverted skin still has to be brought down below the pubic bone to be in the proper position and this is done by cutting and pulling. Some of the scrotal skin is used to fashion what will resemble the outer lips and the excess is discarded. The carefully preserved urethra, sticking up with its catheter in the center of the new vagina, is then amputated at an appropriate length. It is pulled through a buttonhole opening made in the vagina and stitched in place.

Since skin has a natural tendency to contract, surgically constructed vaginas have a tendency to close down. This is counteracted by plastic moulds of varying sizes which are used to dilate the vagina and maintain the appropriate vaginal size. Daily dilatation is mandatory at first. Eventually, finger dilatation is sufficient to maintain adequate vaginal size.

There are a number of complications associated with the male-to-female sex-change operation. Immediate complications include internal blood collection, wound infection, infection of the pubic bone, and a hole between the urethra and the vagina. Delayed complications include narrowing where the urethra was sewn to the skin, urinary tract infection, prostatitis, and closing down of the vagina.

The results can also be cosmetically undesirable: the scrotal labia may be too scanty or too redundant; the urinary opening may be placed too high, causing havoc with urination; the labia and the vagina may be poorly aligned. Finally, even when the results are pleasing to the surgeon, they may not live up to the expectations of the patient.

Female-to-Male

Fewer women than men are openly transsexual. It may be that the transsexual problem occurs with equal frequency in the sexes, but remains more covert with women. Perhaps women realize that the surgical challenge is more difficult and more likely to fail in the female-to-male conversion.

To date, doctors have attempted to fashion a penis from tubed flaps taken from the abdomen, and to fashion a scrotum from the labia. Creating a continuous urinary channel from the natural opening through the new penis has proven a formidable task. And even with the implantation of a penile and testicular prosthesis, there is no sexual sensation in the surgically constructed penis. Most doctors have abandoned this sex-change operation.

I have encountered a number of transsexuals in my practice, but I have never done a sex-change operation. The hospital where I work has decided not to become involved with this health problem and its stance is not unique. The hospital argues that a success rate of one in three is not good enough; that there is an alarming rate of suicide, depression, and psychosis, even after successful surgery.

A friend of mine who used to do sex-change operations at another hospital has abandoned doing them. He says he couldn't handle the constant calls, the veiled threats, the persistent complaints.

I have had some revealing encounters with the transsexual population. I remember asking a patient, waiting to have his procedure done in New York, how he would manage to find the funds to pay for the operation.

"I work as a prostitute," he replied.

I was baffled and showed it. Estrogen had given him the body contours of a female, and with makeup and a dress, he could easily pass for a nice-looking woman. But he still had a penis, scrotum, and testicles.

"Oh, I warn my customers," he said. "Some men are turned off, but most of the clients are curious to know what I can offer."

One transsexual wanted her surgery revised. I examined her and was most impressed with the cosmetic results. And I told her so.

"What could be the matter?" I asked.

"He didn't chop enough off," she said. "When I make love, I still get an erection, and it hurts me and it hurts my partner."

I told her that she was lucky, that next time she could end up with an infection, internal bleeding, or narrowing of the opening.

"But I can't go on like this, it hurts too much," she pleaded. So we arranged a revision. But she has already canceled twice, and I will not be displeased if the surgery never comes to pass.

Another transsexual needs a revision where the vagina made of large bowel meets the skin. The opening is so small it does not allow evacuation of the mucus. I do not anticipate much problem correcting this, but I wonder if she will keep the appointment.

Sex changes in average, everyday life are complicated enough to deal with. I do not envy the transsexual who feels trapped inside the wrong sex. Neither do I envy the surgeon who attempts to make the transsexual's flesh correspond to his or her psychic need.

QUESTIONS AND ANSWERS

Can my partner be allergic to my sperm?
It is uncommon but possible. I treated one woman who broke out in hives whenever her husband didn't use a condom. An immunochemist was very interested in investigating what component in the semen made her allergic, but once the hives were cured by an antihistamine pill taken orally before sex, the patient left the study.

Is it possible that my penis is shriveling up and disappearing?
The penis can become smaller when the male hormone level drops to castrate level, such as after surgical removal of the testicles. More often, however, the "shrinkage" of the penis is simply an overgrowth of adjacent fat tissue. The appearance is more apparent than real.

Can an amputated penis be sewn back on?
Delicate microsurgery can rejoin an amputated penis, but erection will not recur.

Why do people have such a negative attitude about masturbation?
There is a strong tradition in Western civilization condemning pleasure without purpose. Such pleasure is even said to contravene the will of God. Medical science has known for some time that mas-

turbation causes no bodily harm, but only in recent years has it publicized this fact.

Should all menopausal or postmenopausal women take replacement hormones?
Menopausal or postmenopausal women should consider hormone replacement therapy, with the exception of women in the following situations:
1. Women with known or suspected tumors of the type which thrive on estrogen, such as certain breast cancers
2. Women with vaginal bleeding of an unknown origin
3. Women with clots in the vein or with a tendency to thrombophlebitis

Women in the above circumstances should not have hormone replacement therapy. As well, women who have gall bladder disease, jaundice, liver disease, a fibroid in the uterus, hypertension, or fibrocystic disease of the breast should, if they consider hormone replacement, do so with caution.

In almost all other instances hormone replacement therapy can be considered:
1. To reverse the annoying symptoms of hot flashes
2. To counteract the development of atrophic vaginitis and urinary symptoms
3. To counter the inevitable thinning and weakening of bones (osteoporosis)
4. To reduce the possibility of psychological problems such as depression

Of course, hormone replacement therapy is not advised for women who don't need it and inappropriate for those who consider it unsafe.

If your partner is menopausal or postmenopausal and hormone replacement therapy has not been considered, it should be.

Is there any other treatment for women who suffer hot flashes than replacement hormones?
Bellergal tablets, containing the sedative phenobarbital; ergotamine, a drug that counteracts the sympathetic nervous system; and belladonna, a drug that counteracts the parasympathetic nervous system, have all been tried with some success. Clonidine, a pill used to treat high blood pressure, in a dosage that would be ineffective

for hypertension (0.05 milligrams twice daily) has reduced the frequency and severity of the flushing attacks. Progesterone (Provera), at a dosage of twenty milligrams per day, has also been used to treat hot flashes. However, the results from these preparations are not as consistent as the results obtained with hormone replacement therapy.

Why aren't you worried about estrogen in replacement hormones since you worry about estrogen in contraceptive pills?
Hormone replacement in menopausal women attempts to replace what the body no longer produces. Contraceptive pills attempt to distort normal female hormone levels so that a normal body process, ovulation, does not occur.

The dosages of estrogen in replacement hormones are significantly different from the dosages in contraceptive pills. An appropriate hormonal regime for the menopausal woman is 0.65 milligrams of the estrogen Premarin for the first twenty-five days of the month, and five milligrams of the progesterone Provera for days sixteen to twenty-five. A woman taking contraceptive pills, on the other hand, would be taking five to twelve times this amount of estrogen each month.

Can a man who has had a sex-change operation have a baby?
It is theoretically possible to implant an embryo inside a man, administer hormones to simulate pregnancy levels, and thus have a male transsexual carry a baby. There has been a case of a woman, without a uterus, who had a baby. The embryo and its placenta grew on the abdominal wall. But men do not have ovaries, so such a pregnancy would require daily monitoring of hormone levels. Theoretically, a pregnancy is possible, but in reality it does not happen.

Has there ever been a successful female-to-male sex change?
Isolated cases of patients who are pleased with their decisions have been reported. But a result that is cosmetically, functionally, and sexually satisfactory has yet to occur.

10 WOMEN

Throughout the ages, men's private parts have been inextricably connected to those of women. Whatever the impulse—evolutionary, sociological, or simply sexual—men and women often come in pairs. It is not surprising, then, that women's private parts affect the rhythm and cycle of men's lives. And yet most men are in the dark about how women's bodies work. Like Professor Higgins in *My Fair Lady*, they wonder, "Why can't a woman be more like a man?" But women are anatomically and hormonally different from men. If you are going to love them, it's a good idea, at the very least, to know how they work physiologically.

THE DESIGN QUESTION   Women are susceptible to urinary infections because of the design of their urethra. If women could empty their bladders through the belly button as originally designed, it would dramatically reduce female urinary infections. But the original tube from the bladder to the belly button is closed off and is replaced by a urethra, which drains the bladder from below. Women now have a urethral opening just above the vagina.

A woman's urethral tube is as sensitive and as delicate as the lining of the nose. It runs alongside the vagina, which is as tough as leather and as pliable as a rubber band. Its opening is only inches away from the anus. Because it is easy for bacteria to travel, the proximity of the urethral opening to the vagina and the anus creates sex-associated bladder infections. Bacteria travel from the vagina or the anus to the urethra. Foreplay and the thrust of intercourse often

144

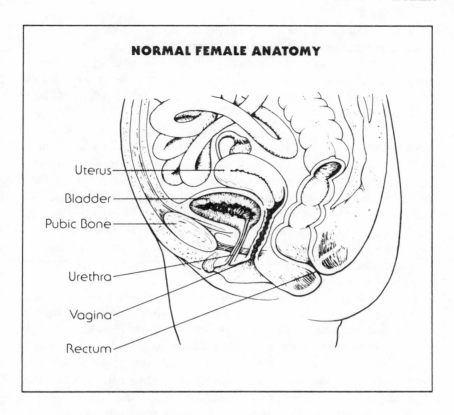

NORMAL FEMALE ANATOMY

Uterus

Bladder

Pubic Bone

Urethra

Vagina

Rectum

milk the bacteria that are in the urethra into the bladder, where urine provides a good medium for bacterial growth. Bacteria make up fifty percent of the dry weight of stool, and these bacteria are the most common cause of urinary infection.

Consequently, men should be careful not to put fecal bacteria into the urethra. During foreplay, a different finger should be used when touching the urethra or the anus. During cunnilingus, the tongue should stop before touching the anus. Harsh manipulation of the area around the urethral opening can cause painful trauma. In general, remember that the urethra is a delicate structure and that fecal bacteria, although microscopic, can still cause painful urinary infection.

Male considerateness during intercourse will reduce female urinary infection, but not eliminate it. In women prone to bladder infection, bowel bacteria actually live on the vulva adjacent to the

145

urinary opening. Women less prone to bladder infection seem to have a protective mechanism that prevents bowel bacteria from "colonizing" this area. In any case, about a quarter of all women between the ages of twenty and forty will have at least one episode of the bladder infection called cystitis, and eighty percent of these will have more than one episode.

HONEYMOON CYSTITIS In most cases of "honeymoon cystitis" intercourse is the direct cause. Why some women are more vulnerable to this problem than others is not clear. It is not simply a matter of hygiene, although a habit such as wiping forward with toilet paper, instead of wiping backward from the vagina to the anus, could be a contributing factor. It is simply, as I have said, that some women have better defense mechanisms than others and their immune systems destroy the bacteria which persist in others.

In diagnosing cystitis it is important to know what kind of bowel bacteria is responsible in order to know what medication to use. This is ascertained by a midstream urine culture. Hospital bacteria are very hardy and resist the usual antibiotics. They must be treated by powerful antibiotics administered directly into the bloodstream, or by injections into a muscle—depending on the results of elaborate laboratory testing. Urinary infection acquired in the community, on the other hand, can be eradicated by most antibacterial pills, and laboratory testing, although helpful, is not essential. The traditional ten- to fourteen-day treatment is being replaced by a shorter drug regime of three to five days; and even a one-shot six-pill dose is being tried with good results, using drugs such as the trimethoprim-sulfamethoxozole combination, or the penicillin type amoxicillin. A shorter regime assures that the complete dosage will be taken: a major problem with the traditional treatment has been that women stopped taking the drug the moment they felt better.

The traditional treatment offered women with cystitis was a course of antibiotics and instructions to empty the bladder immediately after intercourse, like flushing a toilet after use. Infections continued to recur with this regime, and recently we have learned why. Bacteria that cause cystitis adhere to the wall of the bladder and flushing is not sufficient to eliminate them.

I instruct my patients to swab an antiseptic, such as providineiodine, on the vulva daily, to suppress the normal bacterial flora. In addition, I prescribe an antibiotic pill, such as nitrofurantoin (fifty milligrams), to be taken a half hour before intercourse. It may be taken, instead, after intercourse, although that is not as effective. I am impressed by how effective this simple regime has been.

One woman whom I counseled as indicated replied, "You mean I must take the pill every time I make love?"

"Yes."

"Seven times a day."

"You're joking."

"I'm not. This is a relationship that just started and it's going great."

(I still think she was pulling my leg.)

Nitrofurantoin has been my favorite drug, but almost any antibiotics or antibacterial preparations can be substituted. I choose nitrofurantoin because it specifically targets the urinary tract and is less likely to cause side effects or to develop bacteria resistant to the drug. An occasional patient experiences stomach upset and cannot take this drug, and a very rare patient may develop scarring in the lung.

URINARY INFECTIONS— PREGNANCY, POSTMENOPAUSE Silent, or asymptomatic, urinary tract infections occur in six percent of all pregnant women. Untreated, forty percent of these women will develop symptoms and clinical infections of the kidney, whereas none of the treated women will develop symptoms of illness. It is a good idea to culture the urine of pregnant women on a regular basis, perhaps once a month.

Urethral problems and bladder infections are common in postmenopausal women. The lower estrogen level causes the walls of the vagina and urethra to be drier and thinner. Injury and irritation from intercourse become more likely as a consequence. Men whose partners have dry and easily irritated vaginas may help solve the problem with water-soluble lubricants such as Lubafax or K-Gel. Water-insoluble lubricants such as Vaseline or mineral oil can cause a reaction and should not be used.

If the urethra gets irritated, it may scar and the scars may interfere with normal evacuation. And if the bladder is partially blocked by

147

a scarred urethra, it won't be able to empty completely and will be more prone to infection.

When the bladder becomes infected because of urethral scarring, it is helped by periodic dilatations of the urethra and long-term, low-dose antibacterial treatment, such as nitrofurantoin (fifty milligrams taken daily, for several months). If your partner is subject to this problem, she should be offered replacement hormone therapy, using both estrogen and progesterone preparations, as discussed in the section on menopause. As it is usually the gynecologists who prescribe the hormones and the urologists who dilate the urethra and prescribe the antibiotics, the complete treatment, requiring both antibiotics and hormones, is frequently mismanaged.

Often, because the gynecologist sees no gynecological necessity, my patients have not been given replacement hormones. I have, therefore, begun prescribing a course of 0.625 milligrams of the estrogen Premarin for the first twenty-five days of the month, and five milligrams of the progesterone Provera for days sixteen to twenty-five. I use the antibiotic to cure the infection and the hormones to curtail recurrence. I tell my patients that they may talk it over with their gynecologists, but that if there are any objections, I would like to know. I am impressed with my patients' improved health, but concerned by the headaches experienced by a few. In these cases, reducing the hormone dosage to half has eliminated the headaches, but whether or not it will continue to improve the resilience of the vagina and urethra remains to be seen.

The Unstable Bladder
It is possible that your partner may have symptoms of infection—a frequent, urgent desire to urinate and discomfort in the lower abdomen—and have no infection at all. This is a common occurrence. Bladders develop bad habits rather quickly and easily. Thus frequent and urgent urination, originally due to bacterial infection, may persist long after the irritating bacteria have been eliminated. Also, frequency and urgency that began with a stressful life crisis may persist long after the stresses have been resolved. This frequent and urgent desire to empty the bladder, even when there are no bacteria in the urine or disease in the bladder wall, is called an unstable bladder.

148

I believe that our misconceptions about the nervous system contribute to our poor management of this condition. From the first mention of the nervous system, perhaps in high school, students learn that there are two nervous systems—the voluntary and the involuntary. We learn that we can direct a finger here or there because the muscles that guide the movement are directed by the voluntary nervous system. At the same time, we learn that organs such as the bladder are controlled by the involuntary nervous system. Apart from controlling the sphincter muscle and shutting off the flow when we have to, we are taught that the organ behaves autonomously, automatically. Thus when the bladder develops a pattern of emptying too frequently, we cannot understand how we can use our minds to will the organ to change its behavior. Many doctors, as well, are not so certain that the bladder is subject to willpower alone. Thus pills are prescribed to relax the contractions of the bladder muscles. And yet many patients have controlled an unstable bladder without drugs. They have methodically stretched the time intervals between micturition by perhaps five-minute increments every day. Over a period of months, this retraining has had as good results as drugs. Oriental civilizations, it seems, do not have this hangup about the autonomic nervous system. Zen and yoga are fancy names for saying nothing more than this: "Yes, you can control your involuntary nervous system." Of course, it is easier to prescribe a few pills or even psychotherapy.

If the patient has an unstable bladder and cannot voluntarily repattern the frequent and urgent need to urinate, the condition can normally be cured in two months by drugs. The most commonly used drug for this purpose is oxybutynin, at a dosage of five milligrams twice a day. A very dry mouth and throat are inevitable side effects of this drug. When side effects prohibit the use of oxybutynin, I try my patients on flavoxate (Urispas), which is a drug that can relax certain muscles, or dicyclomine hydrochloride, which is an antispasmodic preparation used primarily for an overactive intestine.

HYSTERECTOMY Surgical removal of the uterus is a procedure decided upon by gynecologists, and as a urologist, I have no quarrels with that. But when a hysterectomy is proposed, not because of any malady within the uterus, but because

149

it may help correct urinary symptoms, I do protest. A large uterus may appear to be pressing on the roof of the bladder, but this seldom, if ever, causes urinary symptoms.

There is, also, a tendency to do what are thought of as "preventative" bladder operations at the same time as a hysterectomy. Although hysterectomy can damage bladder and urethral supports, surgery should only be undertaken when there is an actual problem.

Hysterectomy does not necessarily affect the sexuality of most women. But some women find that orgasms become less pleasurable after removal of the uterus. Since we know that pelvic muscles contract and the uterus changes shape and position during sexual excitement and orgasm, it makes sense that the sexual experience in a woman without a uterus may be altered.

If your partner has had a hysterectomy, she may feel psychologically wounded. Extra kindness and consideration at this point will help restore normal sexual feelings.

Stress Incontinence

Stress incontinence is a frequently unmentioned, late complication of hysterectomy. Many doctors choose not to warn patients about this development because the incontinence may only come on years after surgery (although it is the loss of bladder supports during surgery that eventually creates the problem). In addition to women who have had a hysterectomy, this incontinence mostly affects women over fifty who smoke a lot, are overweight, and have had more than two large babies. Kegel's exercises, which control the sphincter muscles, prevent stress incontinence and treat the early cases. The patient is directed to try to stop the urine in the middle of the flow, or at least to slow it down. If she can do that, she is contracting the right muscle. Another instruction is to ask the patient to pull the buttocks together. She is instructed to contract the sphincter muscles one to two hundred times a day. As well, I might ask women to try to squeeze down on my fingers at the time of the examination. A surprising number of women have difficulty comprehending the instruction, many bearing down as if to force a strong flow. Women who can clamp down on the fingers are asked to exercise the muscle for a fifteen-minute period every day. Mild cases, or patients who are very anxious to avoid surgery, are placed on a regime of exercises and medications. The two pills that have proven useful are imipra-

mine, which is an antidepressant, and decongestants such as pseu-
doephedrine. These medications act on nerve receptors located at
the neck of the bladder. The muscle tone increases and resistance
to outflow is increased.

SEXUALITY AND
URINARY CONTROL
Some women cannot achieve orgasm without urinating. I have been consulted a number of times for this "problem." My advice
over the years has been to protect the mattress, nothing more.

One young lady came to see me because she was still bed-wetting
at age twenty-five. She had just gotten engaged and the marriage
date was fast approaching. Was there a way, she asked, that she
could correct the embarrassing problem before the wedding night?
She was free of infection and had no other problems. I prescribed
imipramine, the drug used for mild stress incontinence and bed-
wetting in children; but I warned her that it was unlikely there would
be sufficient time before the wedding for the drug to take effect.

"If you wet the bed on your wedding night," I suggested, "tell your
husband that his sexual prowess and your ecstatic orgasms are responsible."

On the first day of her honeymoon she called to say, "It worked,"
and hung up. To this day I am not sure what worked: the medication
or the story.

My counsel in this case was an unusual solution to an extreme
problem. I do not generally recommend subterfuge. I believe in a
straightforward, honest approach to private part problems. There
is a fundamental difference in the anatomy and physiology of the
two sexes, and I think men and women benefit from knowing the
kind of health problems each may develop. Understanding gives us
an added appreciation of the other and lessens misunderstanding.
Obviously the person who knows about his or her mate's health
makes a better partner.

QUESTIONS AND
ANSWERS
Can a dipstick test be used instead of a
urine culture to test for a bladder infec-
tion?
The dipstick can provide considerable information if the urine sample is fresh and read exactly one minute after dipping. It tells whether
the urine is acid or alkaline, if there is any sugar, protein, red blood

cells, white blood cells, or ketones. The presence of nitrites on the stick is indirect evidence of infection. It is a good first test. But the urine culture is needed to know how infected the specimen is and what specific antibiotics are required.

If I walk on a cold cement floor, can that bring on a bladder infection?

Chilled feet, exposure to a cold draft, and constipation are all clinically recognized as factors that have predisposed the bladder to infection. Why this occurs is not clear.

If I keep using antibiotics for my chronic bladder infection, will I hurt my body?

An allergy to a medication can develop at any time. Symptoms include dizziness, headaches, upset stomach, abdominal cramps, and skin rash. Allergies may also effect changes in the blood picture, and are suspected in cases with a lowered white-cell count or a lowered platelet count. Also, some bacteria adapt to and thrive on a particular antibiotic. Despite these risks, repeated long-term use of antibiotics does alleviate a chronic problem and is usually not dangerous.

Can I harm myself by urinating only once or twice a day?

Some people have naturally large bladders and do not need to evacuate often. But those who develop very large bladders, by not responding to the call of nature, can harm the bladder by overstretching it. This leads to nonresilient bladder muscles that have lost their ability to contract. So lax are some muscles that some women (and very rarely men) can only evacuate the bladder by self-insertion of a catheter several times a day.

Can a woman get bladder symptoms because of menopause?

A young vagina is about thirty cells thick, while an older vagina may thin to about six cells deep. If the older vagina is dry, sore, and itchy, as well as thin, it is suffering from atrophic vaginitis. These vaginal changes do not cause urethral or bladder irritation, but similar changes occur in the urethra and can cause symptoms. These vaginal and urethral changes are largely due to a lack of estrogen and can be reversed by replacement hormones.

152

Can a person get a bladder transplant?

A bladder transplant from one person into another is never done because a new bladder can be made from parts of the small or large intestine. It is a major undertaking, but can be quite successful.

If a woman has surgery to correct stress incontinence, will it affect her sexual enjoyment?

Surgery to correct stress incontinence applies stitches to the so-called G-spot, located on the front wall of the vagina, about four inches from the outside. This area is not scientifically established as a female erogenous zone, but even if it were, sensation should not be affected since the nerves are not damaged in surgery.

What is a partial hysterectomy?

Surgical removal of the uterus without removal of the cervix is called a partial hysterectomy. This operation was done with the intention of reducing damage to the ureter and bladder. Now doctors feel that no woman should consent to a partial hysterectomy as it leaves behind the cervix, a tissue that is prone to cancer formation.

Can a woman have a hysterectomy through the vagina rather than through the lower abdomen?

A woman can state her preference, but the choice is often dependent upon the shape of the pelvis and/or the condition of the uterus.

Pelvises can be wide-necked or narrow-necked. If the pelvis is wide-necked, a vaginal hysterectomy is possible. If the pelvis is too narrow, doing the hysterectomy through the vagina can be damaging to the urinary tract.

If a hysterectomy is being done for cancer of the uterus, then a lymph-node dissection is necessary to stage the disease. In this case, an abdominal hysterectomy is the only choice.

Should a woman get a second opinion if a hysterectomy is proposed?

Hysterectomies are done routinely for the following valid reasons:
1. Cancer of the uterus, ovaries, or vagina
2. Life-threatening hemorrhage during childbirth
3. Prolapse of the uterus, such that it is protruding from the vagina

4. Uncontrolled bleeding associated with a benign tumor of the uterus, called a fibroid
5. Occasional cancers or life-threatening infections that have spread to the uterus

A second opinion should be sought if a hysterectomy is proposed for any other reasons than those listed above.

11 HOW TO TAKE CARE OF YOUR PRIVATE PARTS

Health problems, like divorces, are not matters that people think out beforehand. Thus when a problem arises, even intelligent, well-organized people become frightened and make hasty, irreparable decisions. This reaction is compounded when the health emergency imposes concerns affecting the groin and genital area. Your readings in this book have made you familiar with the workings of your genital system and the problems that can arise. This chapter will introduce you to the health care industry so that you can make appropriate medical decisions.

THE FAMILY DOCTOR   The basic first step is to feel comfortable with your family doctor. You have to be able to talk with him or her, if you want to. A pedantic worrier may be the right doctor for one individual and a confident father figure more appropriate for another. You may not feel comfortable with a doctor who acts as a first aid station and sends all his patients to different specialists. On the other hand, you may feel that your doctor assumes too much responsibility and doesn't refer patients to appropriate specialists soon enough. You may want to talk things out in detail with your doctor, or you may prefer to know only what is necessary. Whatever your choice, your doctor mustn't intimidate you. You should feel at ease talking to him or her about what are normally private matters. Since you cannot change the style of practice of a doctor, the wisest thing to do, if there is a problem, is to change doctors.

Once you have found your doctor, make sure he or she is focusing on your health problem. A doctor should be interested in your occupation, but when you tell him that you are an auto mechanic and he has been having a problem with his alternator, you may spend all the time talking about car problems and neglect the real purpose of your visit. There is nothing wrong in making a friend of your doctor, but keep your medical problem in focus.

And be leery of psychological dismissals. It is widely recognized that as many as ninety percent of all visits to family doctors are for stress or emotional problems. Unless the disease is clear-cut, there is a natural tendency for primary physicians to label problems as psychological. Impotency, for example, is easily dismissed as stress- or age-related. But if you are prematurely and unjustifiably saddled with any psychosomatic label, tell your doctor that you don't want your epitaph to read: "I told you bastards I was sick."

THE PATIENT AS RESOURCE
Sometimes people take extraordinary steps to deny a problem that may already be present. I remember a patient who first came to see me because he saw blood in his urine. Tests showed a bladder tumor, which was removed. But the patient knew that bladder tumors are often a recurrent problem and that blood in the urine can be an early sign of the disease. After the operation, he began urinating in total darkness so that he would not see the color of his urine. At the other extreme are patients who imagine every sickness—such as the patient who drinks too much tea, urinates twice in the night, and thinks he has a prostate problem. These extremes are counterproductive. To get the best care possible, what is needed is an informed, level-headed approach.

Your Medical History
The patient is, potentially, a resource with respect to his or her own health care, and patients who are prepared can help the doctor zero in on the right diagnosis and treatment. Beware the doctor who is not interested in your past illnesses, because he is short-circuiting the fundamentals of medical history, as taught in medical school. A thorough doctor takes detailed notes on your body history, which tells him if the health problem is a recurrence of an old ailment, something related to the old problem, or something new and un-

related. He should also consider your family history because certain illnesses tend to occur more often in certain families, which is not surprising since families share genes and experiences.

Keep a list of all past illnesses that required hospitalization—when they occurred, what the diagnosis was, what treatment was followed, and what the outcome was. If you are taking medication for hypertension, it may be causing your impotence. Decongestants may stop you from urinating. Any manipulation of the urethra may be the cause of infection. A family history of diabetes, cancer, or heart disease is significant, as is a history of unsolved family illness. For example, I have seen more undescended testicles in siblings than in the general population and hernias occur more often in some families than in others. A doctor can't help responding to a challenge, so by all means stimulate his intellectual curiosity.

Medications and Allergies
Make a list of the drugs, with their dosages, that you are taking. Don't rely on your ability to describe them, or on your memory. I remember this unfortunate exchange:

"What medications are you taking?"

"I take a pink pill in the morning, then a blue pill, and a white pill every second day."

"Do you know the names of these pills?"

"No, I remember them by the color."

"Can we call your drugstore?"

"I forgot which one I went to; it's on the bottle, but I don't have the bottle with me."

Can you imagine the service such a patient is likely to receive compared to the patient who appears with a carefully prepared list of medications? Unless he knows what you are taking, the doctor cannot begin a new treatment. He cannot risk a drug combination that may be harmful.

A list of allergies is also appropriate, especially in the case of people who have already had a dangerous drug reaction or are prone to allergies. Asthmatic people, people with hay fever, and people who are allergic to household articles or pets are more likely than others to have allergic reactions to chemicals injected for diagnostic tests—such as dyes used to visualize the heart vessels or to outline the urinary tract.

157

YOUR SURGEON   If you have consulted with your family doctor, explored alternatives, and then have decided to have prostate or other surgery, the choice of a surgeon is your next important decision. It is wise to remember that even when you are sick you have options. Just because there is only one urological surgeon in town, for example, does not mean that you are obliged to stay in that town. And even if your family doctor has gone to the trouble of making arrangements for surgery to be undertaken by a particular surgeon in a particular hospital, whom he describes as "the very best," you are not bound by that arrangement. You may not feel confident or comfortable with this doctor; he may have operated unsuccessfully on someone close to you and you may therefore have misgivings. My feeling is that even if they are superstitious, you may be wise to respond to your misgivings. Exercising these options may seem impolite, but having records transferred to another hospital, or another doctor, is the patient's privilege.

Schooling

You may wonder whether or not it is important to find out what school your surgeon attended, or how he stood in his class. Certainly it is true that medical schools such as Harvard or Johns Hopkins have enormous reputations, unquestionably well deserved. But a school or institution earns its reputation through the quality and quantity of its research, not through its teaching of medical students. And a teacher in a medical school is hardly ever appointed because of an ability to teach. He or she is assigned the task on the basis of research published and because somebody has to do it.

An extraordinarily bright student might do best in a name school, as he will be exposed to the latest and newest developments in the different disciplines. An average student, on the other hand, will get little help weeding out the pertinent material. On the whole, smaller schools do the didactic, basic teaching better. My conclusion after seeing a generation of medical students and hospital residents is that the individual factor far outweighs the institutional factor. Often a superior student from a little school becomes a better specialist than a mediocre student from a large and famous school. Furthermore, performance as a medical student does not translate very well into performance as a specialist. Skills, such as the hand-eye coordination necessary in carving out the prostate or three-dimensional perception, essential in difficult cancer surgery, are not something that can possibly be assessed in a medical school program. Bedside manners can be learned, but real warmth and sensitivity cannot.

As a patient, I would not worry what school my surgeon attended, nor how he performed as a student, although he must have the basic credentials.

Credentials
Surgeons become qualified by sitting for state exams during and after five years of approved training. Those who pass become board-certified surgeons; those who don't can still pass themselves off as specialists—being "board eligible." Once a board-certified surgeon has practiced long enough to have a track record of major cases, he may apply for a fellowship, an honorary title. He presents documentation of his cases and takes an oral exam, but at this point, becoming a Fellow of the American College of Surgeons (F.A.C.S.) is rather routine.

Reputation
The reputation of a surgeon within a hospital or a community does not necessarily mean exceptional skills or competence. It may reflect personal charm, affability, availability—even fee structure. Some patients believe that doctors who charged three times as much for a prostate operation must be three times as good. Non-Medicare fees are arbitrarily set, are not governed by any professional or government regulations, and certainly do not reflect services promised or rendered.

The Choice
Neither schooling, credentials, nor word-of-mouth reputation means as much as how the surgeon performs on a daily basis. I have come to the conclusion that perhaps the best way to choose a surgeon is to ask the hospital staff—nurses, anesthesiologists, doctors—who they consider a good surgeon. Who would they choose if they required a particular operation or care? They have seen the doctor in action and under stress and they know the results. There is no doubt that the hospital staff is the final arbiter of a surgeon's skill.

COMMUNITY VERSUS UNIVERSITY HOSPITAL If you are scheduled for major surgery at a community hospital, would you be better off at a large university medical center? The primary consideration should be medical expertise, and the question of a transfer should certainly be considered. If the suggestion is welcomed but valid reasons are offered as to why it might not be necessary, you might be persuaded to stay. The community hospital might, for example, point out that they have performed your particular procedure hundreds of times and that their complication rate is only six percent compared to the reported twelve percent average. In general, this kind of information is reassuring, although I must confess that I have heard doctors lie about figures. I was shocked at a court session once when a surgeon, testifying about a vesicovaginal fistula (a hole between the vagina and bladder), said that he had looked after cases such as this "hundreds of times." I knew that in a ten-year period there had been dozens, not hundreds, of such cases in major American hospitals. When I objected, the doctor reminded me that "we have to protect our colleagues from unnecessary litigations." The incident gives pause for thought.

If, however, the community hospital convinces you that it has the requisite medical expertise, you may elect to stay. Familiar surroundings, friendly staff, proximity to home, better parking facilities, better visiting hours, etc., are less compelling reasons for a choice of a hospital.

There is an old saying that "those who can, do; and those who can't, teach." Reasoning in this way, some patients think that university teaching hospitals have mediocre surgeons. It could be that a busy unaffiliated surgeon might possibly hone his skills more than a university professor who also teaches, supervises research, and does administrative work. But there are two major reasons why I would choose a university hospital for major surgery. First, the justification for any procedure is more strictly controlled. In a community hospital, operations of questionable merit can go unchallenged; in a university hospital, surgical decisions are subject to the scrutiny of medical students, resident doctors, and peers. A hasty or incorrect diagnosis based on poor or inadequate justifications will become a topic of debate, if not of ridicule. Second, I would feel safer in a hospital where resident doctors are in attendance at all hours. When

160

author-surgeon William A. Nolen needed coronary bypass surgery, he chose a university hospital, not, he says, because he thought the surgeon was superior, but because the resident doctors were there around the clock. It made sense to him and it makes sense to me.

PATIENT-DOCTOR There are patients who always complain about
INTERACTION their previous doctor, and I suspect they complain about me when they move on to the next. There are patients who are never critical of any doctors and patients who are forever fearful. There are glum patients, and there are cheerful patients—a doctor's delight. Doctors are human and are likely to be nice to people who are nice to them. As well, doctors are professionals and appreciate it when a patient is helpful in diagnosis and cooperative in treatment.

I must confess that I get annoyed when patients cannot give me a straight answer to a simple question:

"How many times do you have to empty your bladder during the night?'

"Well, that depends, Doctor."

"Depends on what?"

"How much I have drunk."

"Say, on an average day."

"I have no average day."

"How many times did you get up to go to the bathroom last night?"

"Last night?"

"Yes, last night."

"Well, you'll have to ask my wife that."

"Why?"

"She's more likely to notice that kind of thing."

"Did you get up at all?"

"Oh, yes."

"But you can't tell me how often?"

"Let me see, what day was it yesterday?"

"Yesterday was Monday."

"I think it was Sunday when we had a visit from my brother and his wife. I had some coffee, which I never should have, and I was up all night. Of course, it was all my fault. I didn't have to; I could have declined. But it didn't seem polite; everybody else was having coffee. . . . What was that you were asking?"

161

If one simple question leads to this type of exasperating exchange, the doctor will be totally frustrated by the time he has the full and accurate story upon which he must base ninety percent of his diagnosis.

It is also frustrating when patients do not follow a course of treatment. Consider this exchange:

"I'm not better, Doctor."

"I'm sorry. I was so certain the pills I prescribed would help you."

"Well, I must tell you I didn't take all those pills."

"You didn't?"

"The last time a doctor gave me pills to take, I got so sick. I was afraid it might happen again. I took half a pill for a few days. It didn't make me better, so I stopped."

"I'm sorry I didn't impress upon you how important it was to take the pills in the dosage prescribed."

"I'm sure you did, Doctor, but I was frightened. Can we try it again?"

THE SECOND OPINION   After surgery has been suggested, should you seek a second opinion?

In my estimation you should raise the question of a second opinion, if only to test the reaction. If your doctor becomes difficult, abusive, aggressive, uneasy, or seems to be threatened, you should certainly insist upon a second opinion. On the other hand, if your doctor welcomes the suggestion and helps you in every possible way, I might wonder if it is necessary. Most surgeons with whom I work, when faced with a controversial or complicated problem, raise the possibility of a second opinion before it is suggested by the patient. When the question is not raised, it is usually because there is little to be gained by it. Still, if for some reason you lose faith or confidence in your surgeon, make the change. After all, it is your life and your health we are talking about.

People rarely think of taking preventative measures for their own health, although they are careful to arrange immunization for their children against polio, diphtheria, whooping cough, tetanus, measles, and the like. Yet there are measures you can take to safeguard your health.

Hospitals and health care are often governed by secret, unwritten laws. The universal Medicare program under which I practice in Canada, for example, means that doctors are paid for what they do, not for how well they do it. This means that a doctor who does three good circumcisions and two sloppy ones will collect the same fee as a doctor who does five perfect circumcisions. The Medicare system can only count quantity; it does not count quality. Therefore, make sure you really need the suggested procedure and that you have picked the right doctor to do it properly. In the United States, private insurance often means that the doctor gets higher fees when more tests are done. Your strategy in getting good care should take note of that. You can ask your doctor why he has ordered each test and what information each will provide. If he has to justify the tests, he will be prudent. You might also want to explore reasons for the referral pattern. Is it a referral to a golf buddy, or is it based on past results? And it is often wise not to ask for special considerations. When the normal hospital routine is upset, more things can go wrong. I suspect that that is why there are more complications when relatives of doctors are the patients.

POSTSCRIPT   Look after your health. Your overall physical condition will affect the health of your private parts. Don't dissipate the vibrancy you have been given. Rather, take care of yourself with good diet and regular exercise. In general, people smoke too much, drink too much, sit too much, and eat too much, when they know, all too well, that these habits are detrimental to their health. Smoking, for example, causes not only lung cancer but also bladder cancer. As well, it constricts the small blood vessels of the body and can, by constricting the small artery to the penis, cause impotence. It is good practice, especially for the health of the prostate gland, to eat less, particularly rich red meat, and to consume, instead, fish, white poultry meat, fiber, vegetables, and fruit. It is healthy to exercise more and worry less. Keep tabs on your health and keep clear records of any medical events. If you take care of yourself and are a resourceful, aware patient, you are doing the best you can. The medical profession provides a specific scientific resource, but ultimately you must be responsible for you own health.

INDEX

Doctor
for family, 155–56
patient relationship, 161–62
second opinion, 153–54, 162
surgeon, choosing, 158–59
Doppler flow study, 14
Doxycycline (Vibramycin), 60
Dupuytren's contracture, 29

Ectopic pregnancy, 68
Edecrin. *See* Ethacrynic acid
Edwards, Dr. Robert, 75
Ejaculate
bloody or rust-colored, 5
volume of, 5
Ejaculation, 4–5
painful, 5
premature, 4–5
Electrocardiogram, 40
Electrocautery, 81, 119, 120
ELISA test (enzyme-linked
immunosorbent assay), 123
Embryonal cell carcinoma, 102,
107, 108
Endometriosis, 73
Epididymis, 8, 67, 100
cysts of, 98
Epididymitis, 98, 117
Epigastric vein, inferior, 71
Epispadias, 33
Erectile tissue, 3
Erection, 3–4, 22
Erythromycin, 60, 114, 116, 117
Escherichia coli, 58
Esidrix. *See* Hydrochlorothiazide
Estradiol, 72
Estrogen, 55, 68, 72, 75, 143, 148,
152
Ethacrynic acid (Edecrin),
impotence and, 16

Fallopian tubes, 68, 72, 75, 77–78
Family doctor, 155–56
Fiber-optic light, 39, 42
Fibroid, 154
Finney flexi-rod prosthesis, 20

5-fluorouracil, 120
Flagyl. *See* Metronidazole
Flavoxate (Urispas), 149
Flutamide, 55
Foley catheter, 41, 53
Follicle-stimulating hormone
(FSH). *See* FSH (follicle-
stimulating hormone)
Foreskin, 4, 27–28, 34, 121
Fructose, 9, 66, 67
FSH (follicule-stimulating
hormone), 67, 68, 71, 72, 73
Furosemide (Lasix), impotence
and, 16

Gamma globulin, 126
Gamma rays, 53
Gardnerella vaginalis, 129
Genital herpes. *See* Herpes
Glans (head of the penis), 3, 119,
121
Gonorrhea, 114–15, 130, 131
Gram's stain, 115
Granuloma inguinale, 116
Guanethidine (Ismelin), impotence
and, 17
Gynecologist, 69

Hair loss, from chemotherapy, 106,
111
Haloperidol (Haldol), impotence
and, 17
Head of the penis. *See* Glans
Heart attack, 44
Hemophilus ducreyi, 116
Hepatitis
Type A, 127–28
Type B, 128–29, 131
Hernia, 92–93
anesthetic for surgery, 110
Herpes, 120–22, 130, 131
High blood pressure, drugs for
and impotence, 16–17
HIV (human immunodeficiency
virus), 123
See also AIDS

167

Seminal vesicle, 9, 53, 54
Seminoma, 102–3, 106, 108
Sensate focusing, 13
Sertoli cells, 8
Sex-change operations
   female-to-male, 140–41, 143
   male-to-female, 138–39
Sexology, 13
Sex shop items, 22
Sexual identity, 137–38
Sexual intercourse
   frequency of, 136–37
   painful, 4
   after vasectomy, 89
Sexuality, urinary control and, 151
Sexually transmitted diseases
   (STD), 112–31
   prostatitis, 62–63
Shingles, 121
Silastic, 19–20
Sloan-Kettering Cancer Center, 54
Small-Carrion prosthesis, 20
Smegma bacillus, 31
Spanish fly, 22
Spectinomycin, 115
Speculum, 75
Sperm
   AIDS transmission, 74
   allergy to, 141
   count, 66, 77–78
   microscopic examination of, 67
   number required for
    fertilization, 75, 77–78
   production of, 78
   storage of, 77, 111
Spermatid, 8
Spermatocele, 97
Spermatogonia, 8
Sperm bank, 111
Spironolactone (Aldactone),
   impotence and, 16
Steptoe, Dr. Patrick, 75
Sterilization, male. *See* Vasectomy
Stress incontinence, 150–51, 153
Stroke, 45

Suction devices, 22
Sulfonamide, 116, 117
Surgeon, choice of, 158–59
Syphilis, 112–14, 131

Teratocarcinoma, 102, 107, 108
Testicles
   biopsy, 111
   cancer of. *See* Cancer of the
    testicle
   destruction by mumps, 64
   Leydig cells, 8, 78
   male hormone production, 78
   missing, 65
   removal of, 55, 57
   Sertoli cells, 8
   testosterone production, 15
   torsion of, 99–100
   undescended, 101, 107, 111
Testicular vein, 71
Testosterone (male hormone), 15,
   24, 55, 66, 71
Test-tube fertilization, 75–78
Tetracycline, 60, 85, 95, 114, 115,
   116, 117, 118, 130
T-helper lymphocytes, 126
Thiotepa, 120
Tight foreskin (phimosis), 27–
   28, 34
Transurethral prostatic resection
   (TURP), 41, 42
Trapped foreskin (paraphimosis),
   28, 34
Treponema pallidum, 113
Trichomonas, 118–19
Tricyclic antidepressants,
   impotence and, 17
Trimethoprim-sulfamethoxozole
   (Septra or Bactrim), 60, 116,
   117, 146
Truss, 110
Tubercle bacillus, 98
Tuberculosis, 65
Turner's syndrome, 133
Tylenol, 88

Ultrasound, 39, 51, 56, 103
Undescended testicle, 101, 107,
   111
University of Michigan, 56
Ureaplasma, 117–18
Ureter, 73
Urethra, 3, 6, 42, 47, 52, 53, 114,
   115, 119
   cancer of, 32–33, 54
   See also Bladder
Urethritis, 115, 117
Urinary tract infections, 144–48
Uterus
   cancer of. See Cancer of the
      uterus
   prolapse of, 153

Vaginitis, atrophic, 152
Varicocele
   anatomy of, 95–96
   and fertility, 65
   ligation of, 70–71
   pain and, 110
Vas deferens, 9, 65, 78, 89, 99

Vasectomy
   complications, 84–85
   ethics and morality, 79–80
   reversal, 82, 86–88
   sexual intercourse after, 89
   virility, effect on, 89
VDRC test (for syphilis), 114
Venereal diseases, tropical, 115–16
Venereal warts, 119–20, 131
Vesicovaginal fistula, 160
Vibramycin, 117
Vinblastine, 106
Virag, Dr. Ronald, 15
Virginity, 134
Vitamin C, and infertility, 70
Vitamin E, 22, 29
Vulva, cancer of, 34

Walsh, Dr. Patrick, 51
Warts, venereal. See Venereal warts
Western blot test, 125

X rays, 39, 40, 50
Xylocaine, 81